When the "

M000238248

When the "Dead" Rose in Britain

Premature Burial and the Misdiagnosis of Death During the Enlightenment

NICOLE C. SALOMONE

McFarland & Company, Inc., Publishers
Jefferson, North Carolina

This book has undergone peer review.

ISBN (print) 978-1-4766-8274-7
ISBN (ebook) 978-1-4766-4619-0

LIBRARY OF CONGRESS AND BRITISH LIBRARY
CATALOGUING DATA ARE AVAILABLE

Library of Congress Control Number 2022024176

© 2022 Nicole C. Salomone. All rights reserved

*No part of this book may be reproduced or transmitted in any form
or by any means, electronic or mechanical, including photocopying
or recording, or by any information storage and retrieval system,
without permission in writing from the publisher.*

On the cover: a man wakes up after being prematurely put into his coffin
while being watched by an old woman; from 1805
(used with permission from the Wellcome Collection)

Printed in the United States of America

McFarland & Company, Inc., Publishers
Box 611, Jefferson, North Carolina 28640
www.mcfarlandpub.com

To the smartest woman I know, my Gramma ANNETTE.
And for my eternal research companion, JEDI.

Table of Contents

Acknowledgments

A project of this size is never done alone. I am grateful to my mentors, personal, academic, and professional, who have walked similar paths before and were able to assist as I journeyed down my own path, which was full of prickles, pitfalls, and forgotten cemeteries. Thank you to Dr. Linda Bogar, who told me at the start of my journey that no one knows my research better than me. This mantra has been recited before every talk, every lecture, every panel. It has become my mantra, and it has been shared with aspiring scholars who were battling with their own insecurities relating to their work. Thank you, also, to Drs. Gregory Pressman, Jason Baxter, Vincent Berghella, and Salvatore Mangione, and to Andrea Braverman, PhD, who believed in my ability to succeed in my chosen field and my chosen topic before I had identified what my version of success looked like. The opportunities that you offered to me helped expand my knowledge base and my confidence in my abilities. I will always be grateful for all of the discussions that we had about my research, my goals, and how to take my research to reach those goals. Thank you to my unofficial graduate advisor, Dr. David McCown. I know that the emails that were sent to you towards the end of my degree started to become a bit frantic in nature, but pulling all the parts of a research topic together to write a thesis—an overview of a topic—in six months or less is a big undertaking. Deciding what to keep, what to save for later, what to discard completely or turn into another project altogether—it is all quite daunting. But having someone there to listen and help corral all of that nervous energy was instrumental in the completion of my Master of Arts.

I also want to extend my heartfelt gratitude to my editing team. There were many people who gave their time, experience, and expertise in order to bring this manuscript to completion. It was little more than an extension of my thesis when I brought it to Dr. Diane Cady for content editing and counsel. Through time and patience, discussions and dedication, we were able to create the draft that was approved by my publisher, McFarland and Company, Inc., and their thorough and thoughtful reviewers.

From there, the tone and flow were reimagined, recreated, and rewritten—twice. Stories to add ... ones to take away. Things to allude to as gifts to readers who are not new to the subject, and topics to describe in detail for those who have never pondered the history of the diagnosis of death. The willingness of my dedicated team to share their knowledge and time was imperative to transfer this manuscript from a colossal collection of intertwined ideas to a narrative connected by stories, theories, and people that had previously fallen to the edges of history. Thank you especially to Barbara Puntin, Dr. Philip Tschirhart, Dr. Tracie Provost, Jim Blow, John-Joseph Bober, Kat Curtiss, and Ken Cohen. Your knowledge, wit, humor, and sarcasm have gotten me through some very long days, where the stars twinkled longer than the sunlight, and where we were all reminded that the sun is a star.

They say that the best part of a goal is the journey. I say the best part of the journey is the friends you make along the way. Over the years, there has been a variety of people who helped create a bridge to help me move from where I was to where I wanted to be. Whether assisting in obtaining sources, or discussing the realities of science, the business of death, dissection, and burial, the science of death, the history of religion, wordsmithing, traveling to cemeteries that are *way* off the beaten path, or cracking the code of centuries-old handwriting, I could not have completed this book without your help. Most especially, I would like to thank Susan and Mark Stewart, Kelly Force, Peter Durham, Dr. Samantha Williams, Delmar Watkins, Mark Waks, Karen Veale, Raven, Paul Butler, Beth Ann Bretter, Jill Howard Cozzens, and Greg Lindahl.

It is rarely easy to be friends with a historian, especially one who focuses on such an esoteric and morbid topic. We tend to want to share things with you. And when one wants to share long walks through abandoned cemeteries or stories of gruesome deaths, the choice is to either smile, nod, and back away or to go with the person and hang on for the ride. Somehow, I have found amazing people who have hung on for the ride. I am lucky to have found them mostly for their kindness in showing interest, humor disguised as sarcastic remarks, and inquisitive questions, and in their acting as adventuring partners who have always pushed me to do better, to look deeper, and to keep my audience in mind. To that end, I want to give a very personal and heartfelt thank you to Erika Morton, Thomas Natoli, Gerri Mahn, Robert Peterson, Chelsey and John Knyff, Lucy Martin, Rebecca Buchanan, Bruce Kollmar, David Kidd, Marcus and Kim Wagner, Matthew Stopard, Roza Anthony, Chaz Bergeret, and Carrie Longacre. I hope that this book is everything that you hoped it would be. Additionally, I want to acknowledge those who attended my talks on premature burial and vampirism at various historical, science fiction, and steampunk conferences and conventions. There is little that is more satisfying than being in front of a group of interested individuals who are inquisitive and knowledgeable about a subject. The continued support of these groups has helped drive my research down paths that I may not have otherwise considered.

I would be remiss if I did not specifically thank my Uncle T, who taught me about trepanning when I was a teenager—complete with sound effects—and told me to seek out further information if I was interested. Without that conversation, my understanding of trepanning would have been theoretical at best. Instead, it helped me connect how medical theory begets medical practice and how those practices affect people. It was such a profound moment that it fused itself into my memory and allowed me to recall the information for curatorial discussions relating to the procedure in two different museums in two different countries.

This could not have been completed without the archivists and librarians who assisted as I took up space in their locations for days at a time, who scanned esoteric documents, and who mailed or emailed them to me when the distance to travel was too great. By doing this, they made it possible for me to gain access to many primary source materials that I would not have had otherwise. Most especially, I need to thank those at the Royal College of Physicians (London), the Parliamentary Archives, the London Metropolitan Archive, the Wellcome Collection, the British Library, the Staffordshire Archive, the Huntingdonshire Archive, the Sheffield Archive, the Norfolk Record Office (UK), the Keep Archive (UK), the Cheshire Archive, and the National Archives (UK). Their willingness to assist me and recommend other complementary documents enhanced my research and my final product in innumerable and undeniable ways.

Finally, many thanks must also be made to my family, who listened as I excitedly shared stories about creepy medical theories, supported my dreams of traveling to abandoned cemeteries, looked at pictures of street corners and open fields that have not been relevant in centuries, and continued to support my academic endeavors.

List of Abbreviations

The Company	The Company of Surgeons
MOLA	Museum of London Archeology
RCP	Royal College of Physicians, also known as the College of Physicians, or "the College"
RHS	Royal Humane Society, formerly the Society for the Recovery of the Apparently Drowned
SoA	Society of Apothecaries, also known as "the Society"

Glossary

Body snatching: The act of taking a body from the grave or coffin to sell to medical professionals and school administrators for anatomical study and dissection.

Burking: The action of killing a person to sell their freshly dead corpse to medical professionals for use in their anatomical dissections. After William Burke (1792–1829), who with William Hare murdered 16 people in Edinburgh, Scotland, and sold their bodies to anatomists.

Entombed: When a corpse is placed in a tomb rather than buried in a grave; this is also called interment.

Grave robber: A person who exhumes a grave or opens a tomb for the purpose of stealing the things inside the tomb. Unlike body snatching, the process of grave robbing is not associated with touching or disturbing the body and is more often focused on looting the commodities that may have been enclosed with the body.

Medical professionals: Anatomists, physicians, surgeons, medical assistants, professors/students of anatomy, medicine, or surgery, etc.

Premature repercussions: The actions that happened after people were misdiagnosed as dead. These repercussions include being prematurely enclosed in their coffin, being prematurely buried in their grave or put into their tomb, and being prematurely dissected.

Resurrectionist: A person who exhumed recently buried corpses to sell to medical professionals and school administrators for anatomical study and dissection.

Introduction

In 1788, the *London Times* published a story about the War of Austrian Succession (1740–1748). Early in the war, Commodore Richard Lestock, of the British Royal Navy, was deployed to provide reinforcements to Admiral Nicholas Haddock's forces in the Mediterranean. During the journey, one of the surgeon's mates noticed that a patient had died, and he ordered that the sailor be sewn into his hammock and prepared for burial at sea. As the hammock was closed, one of the stitches ran through the sailor's nose, causing him to move. The hammock was reopened, and blood was discovered "trickling from the wound the needle had punctured."[1] Gin was quickly rubbed onto the temples of the mostly unconscious sailor and he was encouraged to drink some of it. The sailor was brought back to the infirmary and eventually recovered.

Stories such as this have captivated me for decades. I began studying the history of medicine during the 1990s. At that time, I had an adoration for the medicine and surgery of the American Revolution. After a time, my focus shifted from the American side of the Revolution to the British side. Before long, my interests in the history of medicine settled in England. Particular focus was given to what I considered to be "popular medicine": the places within medical theory and practice that connected academic medicine, battlefield medicine, and domestic medicine. It was during this time that I realized that British theories of medicine were in flux during the eighteenth century. Books that were targeted to the poor and infirm included medical treatments that could be made in the home with easily accessible ingredients. Meanwhile, books that were targeted to academic doctors, anatomists, surgeons, and theorists often included medical techniques based on theories from the Renaissance. These theories were often untested, and the techniques continued to be developed throughout the eighteenth century.

By testing and experimenting, improving upon previous techniques, and identifying new medical and surgical practices, the academic medical community developed the beginnings of evidence-based medicine. At

1

that time, the concept of "evidence-based practice" was in its infancy. If the theory or remedy achieved the intended results, then it was accepted as viable. While it was often understood that a root issue caused the symptoms being displayed, it was also assumed that relieving the symptoms would cure the root cause. Additionally, as initial efforts to gather data and observe the results contributed to the formation of the scientific method and strengthening the practices that followed, many of the early studies were limited by exceptionally low numbers of subjects by modern standards.

Throughout my research, I often came across the term *premature burial*. This term occurred most frequently in books about domestic and academic medicine. In both cases, it was accepted as a common problem but was given little attention beyond that. The term was descriptive and the concept easily understood, so I easily accepted that it occurred due to the lack of understanding about human anatomy and physiology. The concept was even alluded to in the 2003 movie *Master & Commander*, when Mr. Blakeney was awaiting surgery and said, "Old Joe told me that when you die, they stitch you up in your hammock with the last stitch through your nose, just to make sure you're not asleep."[2] As evidenced by the article published in the *Times*, this sort of incident was not only a literary trope.

To understand what England was like at the time when premature burial was an accepted part of life, some reverse engineering was necessary. Primary sources and archival resources may not have described a situation or location as unhygienic, but instead new legislation called for the cessation of dumping human blood and fecal matter or animal blood and carcasses into the street. This was unhygienic. Newspaper accounts of premature burial may not have said outright that a person was misdiagnosed as dead but instead used phrasing such as "buried alive," "was seen to breathe during the wake" or "revived in the grave" to indicate that the person had awoken after the funerary process had begun—or was completed. Therefore, it was evident that the subjects of the articles had been incorrectly diagnosed as dead. Likewise, there were insufficient terms to describe the categories of consequences after a person had been incorrectly diagnosed as dead and the burial process had begun. Steps of the burial process included proclaiming the person to be dead, holding a viewing or wake, enclosing the person in their coffin, bringing the body to the cemetery, holding the funeral, burying the body, and filling in the grave. After the official burial process ended, sometimes the corpse was disinterred by men called resurrectionists or body snatchers, who sold them to the medical community for use in dissections or experiments and to teach classes. In addition to the burial process, including the part played by the resurrectionists, some people were reported as reviving at four specific points:

(1) after they were enclosed in their coffin, (2) after they had been buried in their grave or (3) after they were interred in their tomb, or (4) after they had been disinterred and were in the possession of the medical practitioners. For ease of understanding, I created the term "premature repercussions" to describe these four points which indicated what happened to the body after the person had been misdiagnosed as dead and when they were generally reported as reviving.

Mine is not the first foray into the realm of eighteenth-century death studies. Historians and scholars of death and dying, including Clare Gittings, Ruth Richardson, Elizabeth Hurren, Helen MacDonald, Thomas W. Laqueur, and Holly Tucker, paved the way for my research by developing a cohesive narrative of medical history and detailing how it influenced and was influenced by the laws, scientific conventions, and social practices of the time. Like other scholars, I have been intrigued by crossroads of the scientific and the superstitious in the Enlightenment era. Not only were the medical and scientific communities trending away from the theories that had supported their very institution for centuries, but they were on the cusp of medical advancements that would change the world as they knew it. Most especially, my focus was drawn to the social implications that came from an imprecise definition of death.

Other scholars who have written about medicine and science of the eighteenth and nineteenth centuries have generally focused on legislation, commodification, and the division of social classes and resources. This book differs from those predecessors in a number of ways. First, rather than concentrating on the science of death or sociology and commodification of burial practices, I am particularly interested in the way that definitions of death changed as scientific developments evolved during the eighteenth and early nineteenth centuries. Second, pursuing my own curiosity and hoping to share with others some fascinating historical reports, I examine the reasons that people were misdiagnosed as dead and what happened to those who were still living after they received that diagnosis. Finally, by continuing to examine how history influenced the development of meanings associated with death, I turn towards an examination of contemporary social changes illuminated by experiences of misdiagnosed death in the eighteenth century. In closing, I develop connections between these early death studies and vampire literature of the Romantic and Victorian eras.

Over the course of my research, published, printed, and archival stories of misdiagnosed death were analyzed. Primary sources relating to the teaching of anatomy and physiology and the quest for the definition of death were compared. Upon reviewing the work of other scholars who focused on the history of medicine and the history of death during this era, it was noticed that a true medical narrative that focused on the medical community and the differentiating definitions of death was absent. Toward this end, my research contributes the medio-historical narrative of death studies, with the intent to answer the following questions. How were the awareness of misdiagnosed death and the resulting premature repercussions communicated during the eighteenth century? How did this awareness affect the development of early modern medical theories? How did the theories that were developed influence the early modern definition of death? And how did the medical theories and evolving definition of death affect the social norms of eighteenth-century England?

* * *

One of the issues in writing about such a complex topic was how to place the layers so that the reader does not get lost in the details. Generally, the book is set up in chronological order, with connecting topics throughout the centuries. However, it is unfair to expect the reader to know the complex nature of the medical community and how it interacted with the public in the eighteenth century without, first, providing a sense of the evolution of Western medicine up to that point, especially when the core concepts relate to the incorrect diagnosis of death, people being buried alive, and the belief in the existence of vampires.

The more I considered the outcome of premature burial due to an incorrect diagnosis of death, the more questions I had about the medical community during the eighteenth century. It is often stated that the Enlightenment moved the medical and scientific communities from superstition to science. So I wondered how the medical advancements that were taking place changed how death was perceived and understood. By reviewing historical materials and recent academic research, I traced advancements in anatomy, physiology, and the science of death to unearth a network of consistently evolving theories, which built upon each other with the common goal of preserving human lives. Over the course of the eighteenth century, the academic medical community worked tirelessly to try to identify demonstrable and irrefutable signs and symptoms of death. The goal was both to better record and report the causes of death and also to prevent more people from being misdiagnosed as dead and prematurely buried. From these early studies on death, anatomy, physiology and even general surgery began to be identified as their own fields of study.

Creating a foundation of understanding about the world of medical scholarship during the eighteenth century has been a fun and interesting endeavor. It is difficult to start researching the medical history of the eighteenth century without understanding what came before. What were the prior theories of medicine and surgery? How did the study of anatomy and physiology fit into the larger picture? How did ordinary people view medicine and medical theory, and how did their understanding differ from what was known by academic physicians and scholars? In order to provide some answers to these questions, the first two chapters of this book include a brief overview of the ancient theories of Hippocrates and Galen. They explore how medical professionals of the Renaissance started to change the way medicine was studied, moving away from the theories of the ancient scholars Greek and Roman scholars and providing new information based on empirical research and observation.

Chapter 3 introduces the research of key religious and medical scholars from the seventeenth through early nineteenth centuries. Introducing this here allows to reader to understand the information applied to early concepts of death and provides an explanation of the evolution of these theories, which were predicated on those of the other religious and medical scholars. This chapter does not explore the scholarship of every religious and medical professional who sought to identify the signs and symptoms of life or death or the location of the soul. However, it does provide a robust foundation of the information the religious and medical scholars were seeking—such as the physical location of the soul—and how the joint exploration of this subject resulted in the framework on which continually evolving signs, symptoms, and definitions of death have been built.

Chapter 4 introduces problems that those who studied death during the eighteenth century worked to solve. Specifically, the medical community sought to identify the signs of death and the phases that transitioned the body from life to death. They explored how the accepted tests for death could be improved. They embraced the resuscitative process, which would eventually be renamed cardiopulmonary resuscitation (CPR), and tested ways that it could be used to prevent people from being prematurely buried due to being misdiagnosed as dead.

Chapters 5 through 8 continue to explore the burial process, the use of the corpse as a medical device and a commodity, and how the medical and public communities responded to the awareness that people were being misdiagnosed as dead and buried alive. Chapter 5 explores the treatment of the corpse in multiple iterations. Common eighteenth-century burial customs are explained, as well as how they differed due to socio-economic class. The ways that the medical community obtained their corpses for their medical experiments are also explored. This includes an explanation regarding the role of the resurrectionists, who exhumed freshly buried bodies to sell to physicians, surgeons, anatomists, and students for their anatomical dissections. By utilizing the corpse as their commodity, the resurrectionists became an integral part of the medical community.

Chapter 6 provides a robust history of the Royal Humane Society

(London), which promoted and expanded the use of the resuscitative process. The chapter explores how the resuscitative process differed from previous revival methods which had been used after people appeared to have drowned. Stories are provided to give this new medical technique context, and the opposition to its use is presented. Additionally, I present the first modern statistic relating to the prevalence of premature burial and the other premature repercussions. These statistics were determined by analyzing 200 cases of misdiagnosed death from the eighteenth century that were reported in England. The demographics, mortality, and survival rates of those cases, along with the subsequent premature repercussions (enclosure, burial, interment, or dissection), were also analyzed.

Chapter 7 explores how the research done on defining death and preventing premature burial during the eighteenth century was regarded in the nineteenth century. Concerns regarding these issues continued through the beginning of the century. As medical theories advanced, however, the societal awareness diminished. By the end of the nineteenth century, only a few members of the medical community considered premature burial worthy of attention. The point of view of the late nineteenth-century skeptic is presented. Skeptics of the premature burial applied new nineteenth-century medical theories to the historic accounts of misdiagnosed death. While cases were still reported, the common fear of prior centuries had faded into history.

The social implications of fears of being prematurely buried, resulting in the publication of vampire fiction, are explored in Chapter 8. Sometimes, vampirism was acknowledged as an esoteric part of different cultures. Other times, it was considered to be a mystical extension of religion, especially relating to the effect of the soul on the body. These two narratives blended during the medieval era and continued through the eighteenth century. A short analysis of vampire lore and treatises during the medieval through Romantic eras is presented. Different aspects of the history of vampirism were compared against the medical theory of their respective eras and how death was conceptualized at that time. Tying these facts together emphasized what was misunderstood about human anatomy and physiology. The resulting lack of knowledge created fears about people returning from the dead. By analyzing historical accounts of vampires, I identified five distinct traits of a historical vampire story, which are explained in this chapter.

This book does not contain an authoritative analysis of vampire fiction as it relates to medicine. Rather, it includes selected material where vampire fiction echoed the social and medical situations of England and Europe during the eighteenth and early nineteenth centuries. Both the intrigue and the fears of vampires were echoed in early vampire fiction, which started being published at the end of the eighteenth century. Once the reader understands the historical perspective regarding medical theory and the importance of the church and God, it becomes easier to identify the theories, biases, and traits that were reflected in the literature of the time.

The eighteenth century provides the perfect backdrop to showcase the evolution of thought regarding the definition of death, the advancement of medical theory, and vampirism. The origins of legendary literary monsters do not always lurk in the shadows of figurative speech. Religion, the concept of the Other, and the role of charnel houses in death studies have been explored since the nineteenth century. Additionally, readers have been challenged to confront their biases relating to these monsters and explore alternative perspectives. One such perspective is that the origins of these monsters were literary extensions of the facts and fears about life and death during this era. This was especially noticeable in Mary Shelley's *Frankenstein* (1818) and, later, in Bram Stoker's *Dracula* (1897).

Sometimes truth is stranger than fiction, but often fiction echoes truth. This was the case with vampire fiction of the nineteenth century. Relying heavily on the stories of reanimating corpses, fears of premature burial, and the continually ambiguous signs and symptoms of death, the narration and plotlines of vampire fiction were extracted from folklore as well as the social and medical realities of the eighteenth century. These realities situated themselves in the seventeenth-century theories of William Harvey when it was identified that the blood was necessary for life. They emphasized the concept that a body can appear to be both living and dead. They explored the concept of a body living without its soul. By understanding the social and medical realities of the eighteenth century, the authors made a complex and macabre subject palatable for the audiences of their time. This was a contrast to the medical writings of the century before, which were not intended to be read by those outside of medical academia. The medical tracts were written plainly and decisively, with little care taken to make the information land easily on the reader. By examining the medical books, papers, writings, and archival materials from the eighteenth and early nineteenth centuries and from the vampire fiction that followed, I intend to provide a comprehensive narrative of the social impacts of an ambiguous definition of death.

CHAPTER 1

Foundations of Western Medicine and Misdiagnosed Death

"When the Catholics besieged Rouen, in 1562, Francis Civile, one of the most intrepid gentlemen of the Calvinist party, received a wound which made him fall senseless from the rampart into the town. Some soldiers, who supposed him dead, stripped and buried him with the usual negligence on those occasions. A trusty and affectionate person he had retained in his service, desirous of procuring for his master a more honorable burial, went with design to find his body."[1] As he searched, the clouds shifted, and a moonbeam illuminated a ring that Civile always wore. The servant brought Civile to a local hospital where it was noticed that he was still breathing. However, his injuries were too severe for them to try to save him. Instead, the servant brought him to an inn, where he "languished" in bed for four days.[2] Finally, the servant was able to find physicians to tend to Civile's wounds. With proper care and attention, he began to recover.

As he continued to recover, the town was overtaken. "The conquerors were so barbarous as to throw him out of a window."[3] Luckily, he landed on a dung heap where he lay for three days until he was found and taken to a country house. Once again, his injuries were attended to and he recovered, living on for another forty years.

* * *

The misdiagnosis of death affected people of all genders, ages, and economic classes throughout Western civilization. Even those who could afford the best physicians and medical practitioners could not escape it. The best education and personal experience was limited by the rudimentary medical understanding, theories, and philosophies of the time. The permanence of death was in question from the time of ancient Greece through the early nineteenth century. In some cases, people awoke after they had been declared dead. If those who were prematurely declared dead were lucky, they awoke before or at their viewing. If they were less lucky, they awoke in their coffin while awaiting burial or after being set in their intended final resting place. In some extreme cases, people regained consciousness after their bodies had been disinterred and sold to the medical community for use as dissection-bound cadavers. Despite the best efforts of learned physicians and medical theorists, the proper identification of the signs and symptoms of death and its medically accepted definition was a puzzle that took over a millennium to begin to adequately solve.

The issue of death being incorrectly diagnosed, and the consequence of premature burial, was widespread throughout Europe. These misdiagnoses were largely born of misunderstanding rather than malice. As early as the first century CE, medical scholars wrote about people who came back to life during their burial processes. Pliny the Elder (circa 23–49 CE, Rome), for example, wrote an expansive body of work on his observations about the natural world, including the topics of cosmology, astronomy, physical and historical geography, zoology, botany, agriculture, medicine, nutrition, and the uses of metals, minerals, and precious stones. His writings combined theory with stories of the practical application, so his readers could see how those theories could be applied. However, some of his stories included fictional or exaggerated data. Additionally, his belief in magic and superstition were regularly referenced throughout his work. Despite this, his analyses were considered to be an authority on the natural sciences until the late fifteenth century, when early Renaissance scholars began to disprove his work. Pliny's writing included cases of people who had been incorrectly diagnosed as dead but fortuitously regained their consciousness as they were being laid into their graves.[4] One of the stories that he relayed in the seventh book of his *Natural History* was that of the Roman consul Acilius Aviola who had been pronounced as dead and placed on his funeral pyre. Unfortunately, he regained consciousness as the flames grew around him. Onlookers were unable to rescue him from the strong flames, and he died of the injuries that he sustained in the fire.[5] A similar situation was reported to have happened to a praetor of Ancient Rome named Tubero. The only difference was that Tubero was able to be rescued from his burning pyre.[6] Pliny also relayed a more humorous case about a wealthy man who appeared to have died … until he summoned his servants and informed them where to find the money to pay for his own funeral expenses![7]

A contemporary of Pliny's, the Greek philosopher Celsus (25–50 CE) relayed the opinion of the Grecian philosopher Democritus on the signs of death. Democritus had surmised that physicians were not certain of what the signs of life were or if any signs of imminent death existed.[8] He warned that unskilled physicians might mistake diminished signs of life for death.

This point was emphasized in the story of the Grecian physician Asclepiades of Bithynia (2nd century BCE, Rome). One day, Asclepiades came upon a funeral procession of a well-known, yet unnamed, man in the community. Certain that the man was alive, he pushed to get closer to the body as it was being prepared: spices were placed over the man's limbs and his mouth was filled with a "sweet-smelling unguent" before he was anointed.[9] Upon being permitted to handle the body, he confirmed that the man was alive and proclaimed, "He lives! Throw down your torches, take away your fire, demolish the pyre, take back the funeral feast and spread it on his board at home."[10] Although the family was skeptical of his declarations, they agreed to pause the burial ceremony. Under Asclepiades' care, the man recovered and was restored to life.[11] Celsus urged his reader to understand that there were certain indicators that could look like death to the untrained observer but that skilled physicians would not be deceived. He explained that medicine was "a conjectural art, and that the nature of the conjecture is such that although sometimes it should answer very often, notwithstanding it sometimes deceives."[12] In doing so, he admitted to his readers that mistakes happened when it came to identifying the actual signs of death.

Misconceptions about how the body worked did not only affect the diagnosis of death. Similar misconceptions happened regarding disease as well. From antiquity throughout the Middle Ages, it was commonly believed that disease happened *to the body* rather than *within the body*. Religion played heavily into the practice of medicine, as did astrology and astronomy. The latter two terms were used interchangeably until the early sixteenth century, although they differed slightly. In the second century CE, the Egyptian astronomer Claudius Ptolemy explained that astronomy referred to the movement of the stars, sun, and moon in relation to each other, and astrology referred to how those movements impacted people.[13]

As medical scholars theorized about the signs of death, and worked to understand how astrology and astronomy influenced the human body, they based their research on the humoral theory. Surviving from ancient Greece through the Renaissance, this theory was used to explain illness and disease transmission. It was developed by Hippocrates (460–375 BCE) and was built upon by later physicians and philosophers such as Galen and Aristotle. The prolific, well-respected physician Hippocrates was the head of a medical school on the island of Cos, Greece. His contemporary, Plato (428–347 BCE), considered him to be the living representation of Asclepiad, the God of healing in both Greek and Roman mythology.[14] Theories that were once attributed to Hippocrates, personally, are now believed to encompass the theories that were developed within his school. They were recorded in more than 70 books, which were published over a period of several centuries and changed the trajectory of medicine.[15] From this work, Hippocrates earned the honorary title "The Father of Medicine."

The theories of Hippocrates' school contrasted with the commonly held belief that disease was caused by running afoul of the Gods. Instead, these theories set new parameters through which medicine could be viewed and practiced. Disciples of Hippocrates expressed the philosophical belief that medical practitioners were separate from medical theorists because medicine was an art that needed to be practiced in order to obtain both knowledge of the subject matter and the dexterity to apply it. In *On Ancient Medicine*, Hippocrates explained that diet did not constitute as medicine because medicine "was invented for the sake of the sick."[16] It went on to explain "that nobody would have sought for medicine at all, provided the same kinds of diet had suited with men in sickness as in good health."[17]

With that in mind, it was noticed that certain foods affected some sick people differently than others. In those cases, the diseases were observed directly. These observations brought about the inception of the humoral theory, which speculated that the four elements—earth, air, water, and fire—interacted with the four fluids, or humors, of the body—blood, phlegm, black bile and yellow bile—to create the foundation of everything in the universe. The treatise *On the Nature of Man* explained the core of the humoral theory as the following:

> The Human body contains blood, phlegm, yellow bile and black bile. These are the things that make up its constitution and cause its pains and health. Health is primarily that state in which these constituent substances are in the correct proportion to each other, both in strength and quantity, and are well mixed. Pain occurs when one of the substances presents either a deficiency or an excess, or is separated in the body and not mixed with others.[18]

In addition to influencing each other, the humors also affected different parts of the body. Blood affected the heart; phlegm affected the brain; black bile affected the spleen; and yellow bile affected the gall bladder. By keeping these connections in mind, medical practitioners could ascertain which of the humors had an excess or deficiency and then work to balance them out in order to cure maladies.

After the decline of Greece, medical knowledge was absorbed into the religious based medical practices of Rome. There, it was believed that diseases could only be cured by God(s), although the clergy could act as intermediaries. It was during this time that the Roman physician Galen (129–216 CE) advanced Hippocrates theories by writing over 130 medical treatises in an effort to push medical theory forward. Topics which Galen wrote on included disease transmission, the humoral theory, human anatomy, and how the arteries responded in a living vs. dead body. Since the germ theory, as we know it, was not developed for over another 1,600 years, people were often baffled by what precisely caused and transmitted illness. In a prescient guess at an early germ theory, Galen theorized that seeds lived within the body and were capable of transmitting disease, especially the plague. This was considered to be the first suggestion that disease was transmitted by a force other than the God(s). Galen asserted that physicians, rather than priests, would be able to examine, diagnose, and treat the sick. Over the course of four years, he wrote about this theory in his treatises *On Initial Causes* (circa 175 CE), *On the Different Types of Fever* (circa 175 CE), and in his book *Epidemics* (circa 176–178 CE). Despite the time taken to write his theories on disease transmission via seeds, the bulk of his work continued to reference the humoral theory—even when the seeds of disease theory would logically apply. For example, when he published his commentary on Hippocrates' *On the Nature of Man*, he left out the correlation between his seeds of disease theory and Hippocrates' assertion that "the cause of putrefaction in the air [was due to] an excretion from a sick body."[19] Instead, he chose to add specific qualities to balance the humors that were set forth by Hippocrates.

According to the humoral theory, blood was considered to be hot and moist, while black bile was cold and dry. Likewise, phlegm was cold and moist, and yellow bile was hot and dry. Eventually, every plant, animal, and element that could be used to balance the humors was given a quality. These qualities were more believable than the theory that people became sick from seeds that they could neither see nor influence. In contrast, it was easy to observe certain correlations between the qualities, such as the use of a cold, wet compress to treat a fever would lower the fever. Therefore, the humoral theory presented a way to fight illness with results that could be seen and evaluated. The theories and qualities of the humors continued to be enhanced over the centuries and created the foundation of Western medicine.

Another of Galen's notable contributions to the foundation of Western medicine was his scholarship on human anatomy. Since it was illegal to dissect a human cadaver, he used animals whose features he believed were similar enough to humans for the study to still be valid. He chose to use oxen and pigs due to their round faces and because they had a median longitudinal fissure that separated the cerebral hemispheres of the brain. From his experiments, Galen considered the brain to be the "central organ of the nervous system" and knew that the spinal cord was attached to it.[20] He thought that the nerves were organs that communicated "nervous influence" and regulated muscle movement.[21] He theorized that the principle of motion originated in the brain, traveled through the nerves, and caused voluntary movement within the muscles.

Galen also studied how blood moved around the heart and through the rest of the body. While conducting his research, he noticed that the heart expanded and contracted. This discovery led him to the conclusion that blood flowed from the right ventricle into the left ventricle either through pores in the interventricular septum or, sometimes, from "leaks" in the pulmonary circulation.[22] While Galen's observation on how blood moved through the heart advanced the study of how the heart worked, he was not correct in his assessment. Hundreds of years of study later, it was identified that the heart pumps deoxygenated blood to the lungs through the pulmonary arteries and oxygenated blood returns to the heart through the pulmonary veins.

Through his observations of the heart, Galen also noticed that arteries that had been cut responded differently depending on whether the body was alive or dead. He saw that arteries inside living bodies were full of blood. If the body was dead, however, he noticed that the arteries were empty. From these observations, Galen determined that arteries were vessels that contained blood. This contradicted the commonly accepted theory that the arteries housed air that had traveled from the lungs and through the heart.[23] This was a major step forward in the study of human anatomy. Due to his prolific writing on medical theory, Galen's works joined Hippocrates as part of the unquestionable scholars of medical theory and understanding until the sixteenth century.

Herbal Remedies in the Early Renaissance

From the time of antiquity through the Middle Ages and into the early Renaissance, medicine was largely comprised of herbal remedies. Many of the first medical books published were related to botany rather than pharmaceuticals. By the time the Renaissance had begun, medical practitioners began to doubt the validity of that knowledge. Using his position as a Professor of Medicine at the University of Ferrara, Niccolò Leoniceno (1428–1524) reviewed the botanical texts written by the ancient Roman and Grecian scholars and found that he disagreed with many of them. He believed that Pliny had mistranslated many of the botanical texts and that those mistakes hampered the study of the natural world. In order to correct these mistakes, he collected the same plants and rewrote the book based on his own observations. His resulting writings ushered in a new methodology of studying medicine, which was based on personal observation rather than ancient writings.

Leoniceno was not the only medical scholar who doubted the scholarship of the ancient physicians and theorists and sought to update it. The

Swiss physician Philippus Aureolus Theophrastus Bombastus von Hohen-heim (1493–1541), who later renamed himself to Paracelsus, was also dis-enchanted with the reliance on the ancient medical texts. He chose his nickname in order to indicate that he was more advanced than the Gre-cian philosopher Celsus. Throughout Paracelsus' young life, many schol-ars were still looking for answers to medical questions within the research found in the old manuscripts of the Greeks, Romans, and Egyptian physi-cians, philosophers, scientists, and theorists. Around the same time, sci-ence and medical theorists began to study and discuss how humans fit into the scope of nature. Paracelsus believed that physicians who focused solely on the study of nature were hindered by looking to the past for the future of medicine. Rather than trying to change the way established scholars conducted their research, he sought to change the way medical theory was studied and taught within the university system.

Paracelsus decided that the education that he obtained through the European university system was lacking in terms of hands-on learning. After receiving his doctorate from the University of Ferrara in 1516, he spent the next eleven years traveling throughout Europe, Egypt, and the Middle East in order to learn all he could about contemporary medicine in practice. In 1526, he received his medical degree and then became the municipal physician of Basel, Switzerland. As the municipal physician, he was also granted a lecturer position at the University of Basel. His lectures often included situations that he had experienced while he practiced med-icine abroad, and he advocated for the use of chemistry in medicine. Most notably, he was completely opposed to the practice of the humoral the-ory, including how it affected the body and how it fit into the concept of disease transmission. Rather than believing that the onset of disease was caused by an imbalance of the humors, he had developed his own theory of disease transmission. He believed that diseases happened to the body and were caused by poisonous seeds, which he called "astral poison." Paracel-sus theorized that this astral poison had been exhaled from the stars and fell to the earth, lingering in the air until it was inhaled by unsuspecting humans. It would then lay dormant in the body until the stars moved into a pattern that caused it to react. He urged physicians to pay attention to where in the body a disease started, rather than calculating the humoral imbalance. He believed that the latter practice resulted in treatments that were unrelated to the sufferer's ailment. Instead, he argued that remedies were to be carefully managed in order to treat the disease but not sepa-rate it from the body. He believed that completely separating the disease from the body would kill the person. Unfortunately, his colleagues at the university were uninterested in changing their views on medical theory. After only a year, on St. John's Day, a frustrated Paracelsus staged a book burning and set the standard textbooks on medical theory ablaze.[24] His extreme tactics did not have a positive effect. Due to Paracelsus' vivacious personality, new ideas, and profound disrespect for the ancient physicians and their theories, the university asked him to leave.

Paracelsus ushered in the new era of thought at the dawn of the Renaissance by advocating for the replacement of some herbal remedies with the early pharmaceutical remedies mercury, sulphur, and salt, which he called the Tria Prima.[25] It was his belief that as physicians understood how these three elements interacted with each other, they would be able to cure diseases more effectually. He theorized that since diseases were natural occurrences, their cures would also be found in nature.[26] In the following centuries, this methodology was standardized and became a basic part of the way science and medicine were studied.

In addition to Leoniceno and Paracelsus, other medical scholars who doubted the ancient medical texts were working to change the way that medicine was considered, studied, and taught. The Veronese physician and astronomer Girolamo Fracastoro (1478–1553) was one of them. Building upon the theories of Paracelsus, Fracastoro theorized the foundations of our modern germ theory with remarkable accuracy. He believed that that disease was a type of putrefaction and that as the body decayed it released small, self-multiplying putrefying particles that infected others upon contact.[27] These were transferred either through direct contact, through indirect contact (person to object to person), or through the air.[28] He postulated that airborne diseases acted differently than the others and considered their transmission to be a "mystery."[29] Often it was believed that diseases were caused by foul smelling air, a concept that would later be known as miasma or mal-aria. This was identified because people who had not come in contact with each other were sometimes struck down with the same disease. Unfortunately, the manifestation and transmission of airborne diseases continued to stump medical practitioners and theorists for centuries.

Plague Orders in Sixteenth Century England

In 1518 a plague epidemic swept through England. That same year, King Henry VIII (1491–1547) initiated two "firsts" that would alter the course of how medicine was studied by medical professionals and utilized by the public in England. He instituted the first medical college in England, the College of Physicians of London ("the College" or "RCP"), and he enacted the first plague orders. These simultaneous actions were not coincidental. Plague outbreaks were a semi-regular occurrence in

London, so people became adept at identifying its presence and symptoms. Due to its periodic occurrence in London, the city administration developed the plague orders to regulate the response to more severe outbreaks. These orders delegated responsibility to different city officials in London, the London suburbs, and the further reaching counties. With each subsequent plague outbreak, the orders were updated and modified based on lessons learned during the previous outbreaks. In 1543, the Lord Mayor of London began to disseminate the updated plague orders regulating the city with his aldermen.[30] The aldermen would then ensure that the orders were heeded by the constabulary, examiners, searchers, physicians, and surgeons. By 1574, the plague orders were also distributed to parishes and churches and nailed onto posts as an effort to relay up-to-date information to the public.

Since the plague orders allowed for government oversight of the public health of the area, the College of Physicians was called on to provide their collective knowledge in ways that "could help the monarchy temper the effects of plague."[31] Although the College was founded at a time when medical training was not well regulated, the original members included some of the most prestigious physicians of the time. The goals of the College were to grant licenses to qualified practitioners and to hold "unqualified practitioners and those engaging in malpractice" accountable.[32] Run like an academic collegium, the first president of the College, Thomas Linacre (1460–1524), desired physicians to be considered the most elite in the medical community. Members had to pass examinations and pay annual dues to maintain their license to practice. Those who had graduated from Cambridge or Oxford University also had the ability to become a Fellow of the College. By 1523, the influence of the College was expanded to include all of England. When Linacre died in 1524, he left his home to the College for use as their permanent address. The stone house was several stories high and included a meeting room, a library, and an anatomy theater, which allowed the members to privately practice dissections.

As the College worked to secure its reputation in London and England at large, a structure developed which governed how the different facets of medicine were to be practiced. In 1540, it was enacted that physicians were authorized to search apothecary shops and to practice the art of surgery, thereby validating physicians were at the top of the medical hierarchy. That same year, King Henry VIII incorporated the Company of Barbers and Surgeons with the encouragement of his own surgeon, Thomas Vicary. Initially, the Worshipful Company of Barbers had 185 members and the Guild of Surgeons had around 12.[33] While barbers were responsible for minor surgeries such as pulling teeth, bleeding patients, and lancing and draining abscesses, surgeons were allowed to do more intricate and invasive procedures, such as removing tumors and abscesses, amputating limbs, resetting bones and joints, and cauterizing wounds. The goal of joining the groups was two-fold: first, it was believed that their co-joining would help both groups gain political standing and credibility in the medical community,[34] and second, it was hoped that combining the two groups would provide surgical apprentices with an education in the theory and practice of anatomy.[35] Despite the incorporation of the two groups into one company, they still existed as two separate groups. In 1540, the Act Concerning Barbers and Surgeons to be of one Company clearly delineated the roles of each group and stated, "No Barber in *London* shall use Surgery; or any Surgeon of *London* use Barbery."[36] The act also loosely regulated how the barbers and surgeons could practice within the city of London. For example, only barbers who were part of the Company were permitted to have their own shop within the city. Surgeons were allowed to have their own shop and hang a sign near their door as advertising.

The Act Concerning Barbers and Surgeons to be of one Company went on to say that the bodies of four executed felonious criminals could be taken from the gallows and used for anatomical dissections by the Company annually, in perpetuity, in order to enhance the "Knowledge Instruction Insight Learning and Experience in the said Science or Faculty of Surgery."[37] On February 24, 1565, Queen Elizabeth I decreed that three or four bodies of thieves or murderers who were executed at Tyburn would be given to the College "to be dissorted [*sic*] and anatomized."[38] Both surgeons and physicians were known to wait at the gallows to take ownership of the same bodies to study practical anatomy, especially if the number of people being executed did not meet the amount that each group was entitled to. In some cases, one group would try to buy the body of the criminal before the person was executed. In order to do this, a representative from either group would go to the jail and pay the criminal, directly, for use of their body after death. The number of bodies to be given over to the College of Physicians increased to six under Charles II in 1663.[39] In order to engage and educate the public, the Company of Barber-Surgeons held at least one public anatomization per year. A precursor to the concept of dinner and a show, the Company held an event where the elite were invited to a banquet that culminated with a dissection demonstration. Although the physicians and surgeons found ways to work together, the formal arrangement was tenuous at best. The Company of Barber-Surgeons dissolved in 1745, at which time the surgeons formed the Company of Surgeons. The Company of Surgeons then became the Royal College of Surgeons of London in 1800.

Medical Theory During the Renaissance

Medical theory during the Renaissance was disjointed. Theories were only starting to grow beyond their humoral base. Medical training for physicians, anatomists, and surgeons was not formalized or mandatory. Of the three groups, only physicians and anatomists could attain a university education in their respective fields. Physicians who received a university education had options of how to utilize that training. They could rotate return the academic system and become professors. If they chose to see patients, they were permitted to work in small towns, in large cities, with the military, in hospitals, or become personally employed by nobility or royalty.

While anatomists and surgeons could attain similar education, training, and societal acceptance as physicians, neither anatomists nor surgeons had access to all of them. Anatomists—medical professionals who studied human anatomy and physiology—were slowly becoming accepted by the university system. Dissection of the human body was a relatively new concept that started to gain popularity in the fourteenth century. Previously, Galen's theories had sufficed for knowledge on human anatomy. His theories were perpetuated throughout the Middle Ages, and the four major medical colleges of Europe continued to teach them through the Renaissance. Classes taught to anatomists included the dissection and examination of animals, such as pigs, just as Galen had done. Since students continued to learn the same animal anatomy in conjunction with the texts, the study of anatomy remained effectively unchanged. Although the medical community, at large, was not prepared to challenge the theories of Galen, there were some pioneers who forced Western medicine to evolve.

One such person was the Belgian-born anatomist Andreas Vesalius (1514–1564). Prior to attaining a position as a Professor of Surgery and Anatomy at the University of Padua, he had boarded in the same student housing as the second president of the College of Physicians of London, John Caius. Vesalius' prolific writings and detailed drawings depicting the inside the human body accurately earned him the nickname "the father of modern anatomy." His book *De Humani Corporis Fabrica* (1543) ushered in a new era of anatomical study and included detailed information on bones, cartilage, muscles, ligaments, veins, arteries, and organs. This accurate assessment of human anatomy was obtained by using freshly exhumed human cadavers rather than the bodies of animals. The observation of the inner workings of the human body improved the validity of his research and aided in the creation of new anatomical and physiological theories in the following centuries.

Even as Vesalius discovered that the Galenic texts had anatomical inaccuracies, and taught about them in his classes, he delayed publishing his findings. He understood that the large undertaking of challenging Galen had to be done tactfully in order to be received well by his respected and esteemed colleagues. This point was emphasized in the dedication of *De Humani Corporis Fabrica* where he stated that he expected his work to come under scrutiny, especially by medical authorities who had not yet taken his classes or attended his dissections.[40] In the second edition of *De Humani…* (1555), he explained that he was unable to recreate Galen's experiment on how blood moved through the heart.[41] Although Galen had claimed that blood moved from the right to left ventricle through the septum, Vesalius did not believe that such blood flow was possible. Vesalius handled other instances of disproving the Galenic theories with similar diplomacy: writing with great respect of the prior writings, while still pointing out that they were, in fact, inaccurate in relation to the human body.

A new era had begun in the wake of changing information about human anatomy, physiology, and medicine. The establishment of these new theories created a divide in the medical community. While some people were averse to change and wished to continue to study the ancient texts, others favored the new anatomical and empirical information that was being published. These new theories were used as a foundation for new observations, new analysis, and new theories, which would guide the study of medicine, anatomy, and surgery through next two centuries.

Meanwhile, surgeons were not able to receive formalized training at the university level. Instead, they received training through serving in the military and then opened their own surgeries upon release. If they were exceptionally good at their craft, they could be hired to work privately for nobles or royalty. Surgery was a completely separate field of study from medicine and anatomy because surgeons used tools in addition to the growing anatomical knowledge to fix medical issues. Despite the extra skills necessary to be a surgeon, most physicians still regarded surgery as a type of unscientific butchering. This mindset gave the overall impression that surgery was, at best, a trade and more suitable to be taught via an apprenticeship than through the university system.

Despite the general disrespect given to surgeons, Ambroise Paré (1510–1590) stood apart and brought an air of respectability to the profession. This French surgeon served in his country's army for 15 years, from 1537 to 1552. During this time, Paré used his skills as a surgeon to bring comfort to those who were in his care. One of his most notable contributions to the field pertained to the treatment of gunshot wounds. Normally, these wounds were treated by dipping a piece of cloth in boiling oil and placing it on or through the wound. Although this method of treatment cauterized the wound, it often resulted in infection, pain, fevers, and suffering. Having run out of oil at one point, he treated the wounds with a mixture of rose oil, egg yolks, and turpentine (pine resin).[42] He noticed that those who had been treated with the turpentine mixture healed with less pain and swelling around their wounds. Although the cause was not understood at the time, this was due to the antiseptic properties of the turpentine. This result was repeated by a salve created by another surgeon who also had great success in curing gunshot wounds. After years of trying to gain his favor, Paré finally received the recipe: "to boil, in oil of lilies, young whelps just born,

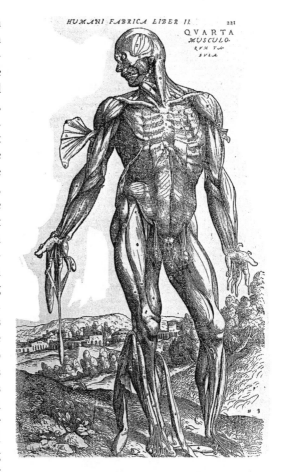

Vesalius' "Fourth Muscle Man." This shows how Vesalius represented human anatomy in his *De Humani Corporis Fabrica* (used with permission from the Wellcome Collection. Attribution 4.0 International [CC BY 4.0]).

and earthworms prepared with Venetian turpentine."[43] Throughout his lifetime, Paré worked his way up from a barber-surgeon to the royal surgeon to the French kings Henry II, Francis II, Charles IX, and Henry III.

Due to the differences in theoretical study and practical application of their subjects, physicians, anatomists, and surgeons worked alongside each other rather than with each other. This was exemplified in 1559 when King Henry II of France (1519–1559) was wounded during a demonstrative joust. Jousting was a martial game which was fought with a lance or a spear against another person while both were on horseback. This particular joust took place at an opulent three-day long festival that was being hosted by King Henry II to celebrate the upcoming marriages of the King's sister, Margaret, and his daughter, Elizabeth. The rules of the day indicated that there were three challenges, and King Henry II faced them all in front of the assembled crowd. During the first challenge, the King jousted against the Duke of Savoy. Although both of them were able to break their lances upon the other, King Henry II was declared to be the winner because the duke's horse had reacted when the lances broke. His next challenge was won against the Duke of Guise. The third challenge was against the captain of his Foot Guards, the Comte de Montgomery, but the King was unhappy with the outcome.

The initial joust against the Comte de Montgomery was successful for King Henry II. However, the Comte had also done well, and his blow nearly unseated the King. Unhappy that he had not achieved a clear victory, the King requested that the joust be refought. Despite being told by the judges, the Queen, close council, and Montgomery himself, that he had won the day, the King insisted that the joust be refought and would not take no for an answer. The outcome of the final joust was certainly more decisive but not in the way that the King had undoubtedly expected. In the new joust, both lances broke again, but this time Montgomery did not let go of his lance. As the horses continued past each other, the broken end of his lance inadvertently raised the King's visor and then struck him in the face, just above the right eye.

The King was immediately brought into his private chamber, where he was attended to by his principle royal physician. After looking at the King's wound, the royal physician requested the presence and assistance of Andreas Vesalius. Since the King had fainted while he was being moved from the joust to the castle, he was "revived with a mixture of rosewater and vinegar."[44] Taking care of his facial wound was more complicated. Although medicine had started to evolve into a science, it was still somewhat rooted in the ancient medical theories. Therefore the solution used was a mixture of older theory and empirical observation. After the splinters were removed from his eye and face and the wound was properly dressed, King Henry II was given a purgative to empty his stomach. When he became feverish, he was bled and rubbed with ice in order to bring his temperature down. When Andreas Vesalius arrived a few days later, he quickly partnered with the King's Surgeon, Ambroise Paré, to develop a plan of care for the King. Vesalius tested for the severity of the injury by having King Henry II bite down on a piece of cloth and pulling on it. When the King cried out in pain, Vesalius became concerned that the wound was not healing. In order to understand the depth of the injury, Paré and Vesalius thrust the end of Montgomery's lance into the disembodied heads of four executed criminals. Through these experiments, they determined that the lance had only pierced the eye and had not continued into the brain. Despite having two of the most prestigious and prolific medical practitioners of the time at his side, King Henry II of France died of his wounds on July 10, 1559. Vesalius' autopsy report stated that their initial theories had only been partially correct and that "many splinters were driven into [the] lateral wall" of the right eye and the socket, therefore "causing a very severe concussion of the brain."[45]

* * *

The U.S. National Library of Medicine is in possession of a sixteenth-century copy of a letter, which explained Vesalius had obtained familial permission to perform an autopsy on the body of a Spanish nobleman but upon opening the chest cavity discovered that the heart was still beating; the nobleman subsequently died.[46] The family called upon the Spanish Inquisition to press charges against Vesalius for murder. Before the charges could be placed, however, King Philip II intervened and ordered Vesalius to go on a pilgrimage as penance for what had transpired.[47] Although this story had been repeated throughout history by medical professionals such as Drs. Ambrose Paré (1579), Jean-Benigne Winslow (1746), and James Curry (1792), it is currently accepted as a myth. Whether the story was true or not makes little difference in this case. The important aspect is the story itself: that the nobleman was declared as dead by a medical professional and then dissected prior to actually being dead. Stories with this theme were recorded during the Renaissance and repeated throughout the eighteenth and into the nineteenth centuries. This proved that the concepts of someone being misdiagnosed as dead, being treated as if they were dead, and dying due to the misdiagnosis were believed.

A similar situation took place during the embalming of Cardinal Diego de Espinosa (1502–1572). An account reported during the middle of the eighteenth century claimed that the Cardinal had been diagnosed as dead and the body was given over to a surgeon to be embalmed in preparation for burial. As the surgeon was preparing to begin, the Cardinal began to regain consciousness and pushed the surgeons' hand away.[48] Nonetheless, the operating surgeon was not deterred and continued with the embalming process, which caused the absolute death of the Cardinal.[49] This story represents one of the earliest reports of a premature dissection and shows a bias against the humanity of the surgeon. Although most cases of premature dissection proved to be fatal, this is the only one in which the operating medical professional continued the procedure even after learning that his subject was alive.

The Renaissance set the stage for the understanding of medicine, anatomy, and physiology that came afterwards. Although his methods were, arguably, excessive, Paracelsus' view on the lack of importance of the humors directed a shift in the way that the ancient texts were regarded academically. Vesalius' opinion that the best way to learn about human anatomy was to study an actual human body helped teach people the importance of doing so. It revealed flaws in the traditionalist texts and set the precedent for future medical professionals to do the same. Beginning in the Renaissance, physicians, anatomists, and surgeons were able to move away from the medical community's reliance on ancient medical theory and start to develop new and improved theories based on empirical data and observation.

Although cases of misdiagnosed death were reported in ancient Greece and Rome, the theory and technology to prevent such accidents from occurring did not come about until the eighteenth century. Medical theory of the eighteenth century was rooted in the major changes that occurred during and after the Renaissance. Expanded exploration by Western European countries during the late Middle Ages caused a difference in thought as Europe shifted into the next era. Factors that helped evolve thought included the introduction of gunpowder into warfare, new trade routes, and the invention of the printing press.[50] Religious movements led to reformations and counter-reformations. The scientific and medical texts of ancient Greece and Rome were reexamined and corrected. All this being considered, it should come as no surprise that a new age of medicine was dawning.

CHAPTER 2

The Function of Anatomy and Physiology in the Seventeenth Century

In late July of 1674, Mrs. Blunden, of Basingstoke, overdosed on poppy-water and fell into such a deep sleep that she was determined to be dead. Those who were closest to her agreed that she had died because they could not determine any "palpitation of the heart, motion of the pulse, breathings at her mouth or nose, nor any sensible warmth to be discerned in the whole body."[1] Her body was laid out to be watched. One observer noticed that when she pressed on her face, the blood seemed to rush there. Additionally, there was a blush in her cheeks. But the weather was hot and her family decided that she should be buried quickly to keep them from having to watch the body decay.

Several people in attendance were skeptical of her family's decision due to the indication that Mrs. Blunden was alive. Additionally, her husband was away on business and would not be back in time for the funeral. However, no one stopped the proceedings. Her body was placed in a coffin and set upon two stools so that people could say their final good-byes before the burial. Another observer thought that both the coffin and the stools started to shake. Uncertain about what could cause such a well-made coffin to move, they assumed that either the stools were unsteady, or people were knocking into the coffin as they passed by. The body was buried without further delay.

The following evening, a few students were socializing in the churchyard and thought that they heard a voice calling from underground, "Take me out of my grave."[2] Terrified, they ran and told their families what they had heard. The story was so unbelievable that nobody took them seriously. When their reports reached their schoolmaster, they were punished for telling lies. Frustrated, the students returned to the gravesite the next day. Again, they heard shouts for release emanating from the grave, and told their school master about it.

This time, he believed the story and followed them to Mrs. Blunden's grave. Placing his ear on the ground, he heard the same as they had claimed. Acting quickly, he sought to exhume the body, but did not have the authority to do so. After the church wardens were consulted, the clearance to open the grave was issued. When the body was exhumed, it was noticed that she had "most lamentably beaten" herself after she had been prematurely buried.[3] However, no signs of life could be discerned, so she was lowered back into the grave. The grave was left open overnight, and people were appointed to stay nearby to see if she would rouse again. But it rained that night, so the people who were supposed to stay with her decided to go home instead. When the body was viewed again the next day, it was found that she had "torn off great parts of her winding sheet, scratched her self [sic] first in several places, and beaten her mouth so long, till it was all in gore and blood."[4] The coroner asserted that her hasty burial caused her death. However, the town doctor assured those assembled that he had "I [sic] a looking-glass to her mouth a considerable time, and yet could not discern the least breath to come from her."[5] He said that he had used this test before, and this was the first time that it had resulted in the misdiagnosis of death.

* * *

The seventeenth century blustered into existence in England. The plague, which had come and gone with relative regularity in the preceding century, had made numerous appearances in the 1590s and early 1600s. Physicians bore the brunt of the social implications of containing it, controlling it, and ultimately curing it. Without a viable germ theory and years before Galileo developed the first microscope, they were combating a disease whose cause and transmission they did not properly understand. The regular updating and dissemination of the plague orders allowed London's city administration to regulate how the city officials could enforce the rules set in place during the plague; however, they could not force the citizens of the city to follow them. Additionally, while London struggled through the plague, the great medical minds of Western Europe continued to further research the fields of human anatomy and physiology. Although the medical community was still divided regarding how much faith to put into the theories of the ancient medical scholars, such as Hippocrates and Galen, seventeenth-century medical scholars were committed to identifying what caused a human to be alive. Particular progress was made in understanding heart and brain functions, how the soul was incorporated into human physiology, and how a person would be affected if these areas worked at diminished capacity or stopped working completely.

Although London was a city of great power and influence throughout the Western world during the seventeenth century, it had not yet become a cosmopolitan metropolis. It was an over-crowded, stinky, muddy mess. Streets were nothing more than glorified trash heaps with refuse from chamber pots, blood that had been discarded by barber-surgeons, innards of animals that had been boiled and butchered, and run off from dung hills mixing with trash, lost items, and mud. The moat that had once surrounded the city walls had long since fallen into a state of disrepair. By the beginning of the eighteenth century, the level of filth in London had become so notorious that Johnathan Swift described it in his poem "A Description of a City Shower" (1710):

> Filths of all hues and odour, seem to tell
> What street they sail'd from, by their sight and smell.[6]

The city center had become so crowded that any buildings built after 1580 had to be at least three miles away from the city gates. There was a decline in the expansion of London, which prevented the creation of new housing in the overpopulated city.[7] Houses were constructed with a combination of stone and wood with thatched roofs. As overcrowding became worse, building upward was the sole option, since they could no longer be built out. This construction resulted in many homes being two or three levels tall, rickety and bent. They leaned over the alleyways and streets, which were so narrow that the roofs touched in some places. As the top of the homes began to lean towards each other, the weight of the upper floors caused the frames to bow and the lower floors to buckle. Each level of the house consisted of up to three rooms where entire families would live with their pets and any barn animals that they owned. Garbage was left in large freestanding piles just outside the doorway and care was not taken to keep the mice, rats, or other pests and vermin outside.

On March 24, 1603, Queen Elizabeth I died. London shopkeepers prepared for the influx of business that was expected from those arriving to see her funeral procession. Merchants arrived from throughout the country to set up temporary structures along the procession route. Thousands flocked to London from throughout Europe to partake in the spectacle. Some of the countries that visitors arrived from, such as Lisbon, Spain, and Germany, recently had their own issues with plague outbreaks. In addition to people, these ships transported rats that carried plague-infected fleas. While it is unlikely that the sick rats would have left the cool darkness of the ships, the fleas could have easily jumped to the warm humans who then proceeded to fill the city's busy streets and taverns. People were so busy preparing for the Queen Elizabeth's funeral procession that it was not noticed when a handful of people died from the plague. Her funeral procession took place on April 28, 1603, and ran from Whitehall Palace to Westminster Abbey.

The causes of infectious disease remained a mystery throughout the seventeenth century. Many still believed that infectious disease was caused by "mal-aria," or foul smelling air emitted from the earth, and was most likely to occur in either overcrowded cities or marsh laden country towns. In cities, the stench in the air emitted from streets, sewers, and moats, which were choked with garbage, hay, and the feces of humans and animals. Country towns that were set near swamps and marshes and cities that were near ports, rivers, and lakes had reports of fevers outbreaks like "marsh fever" or "ague" which have since been attributed to malaria. The onset of plague and malaria mirrored each other, so the inception of a plague outbreak could be easily missed. At the start of both diseases, the person would be stricken with a very high fever, chills, muscle aches, and a general feeling of malaise. As the diseases advanced, however, the symptoms differed drastically. Malaria was exhibited by gastrointestinal issues, such as vomiting or diarrhea. The plague brought on pus-filled buboes which developed on and around the person's lymph nodes. As the body tissue around the buboes died, it became gangrenous and turned black.

The reemergence of the plague, in 1603, transitioned from normal to problematic when it was reported that nearly 100 people died from it in May. The city administration of London met and predicted that chaos was about to erupt. They made the decision to focus on the traffic moving in and out of the city during preparations for the coronation of James I. As thousands of people continued to flood into London, their luck seemed to take an even worse turn when the German astrologer, Johannes Kepler, reported a partial lunar eclipse later that month. Since it was still believed that the movement of the "heavenly bodies" impacted disease *and* there were eclipses that correlated with the end of plague outbreaks in 1551, 1579, 1583, and 1592, it was easy to believe that this eclipse would also have an effect on the plague. On May 26, 1603, the Lord Mayor issued plague orders detailing where and when the administrative councils would meet to update the information that would be distributed throughout the city, calculate the mortality totals from each parish, and organize how city officials, doctors, and citizens were expected to behave. On May 29, a Royal Proclamation was issued ordering anyone who did not have business in London to leave until the end of July. Meanwhile, the death toll slowly climbed over 300 in June.

In addition to providing administrative guidance and distributing remedies to be used against the plague, the plague orders also allowed the city's administration to quarantine houses whose inhabitants had been infected by the plague. London's city administration enacted this effort in July 1603 to control the spread after 3,000 people died of plague. Public gatherings of all kinds were prohibited including attending public houses, taverns, and theaters. A six week quarantine was required for anyone who had either contracted the disease or lived with someone else who was afflicted. In order to ensure compliance, the London constabulary nailed the doors shut and marked houses with a red cross and the inscription "Lord Have Mercy Upon Us," so that others would know to stay away from that house. Those quarantined were not permitted to interact with anyone else or exit their homes for any reason, including getting food or drink, to see their family, or to go to work. The only people who were allowed to leave their homes were farmers, so that they could tend to their lands. While a house was under quarantine, the only person who was permitted to enter was a physician.

The constables also worked closely with the examiners, who discretely ensured adherence to the plague orders and reported which houses had been struck by the plague to the constables. The examiners worked with searchers, who were responsible for viewing the bodies of those who were either infected by or died from the plague. Unlike the rest of London's administration, the searchers were typically older women due to the experience they were assumed to have had from caring for sick family members. The searchers were responsible for reporting the amount of people who had contracted or died from plague to the aldermen and parish clerk. The plague orders indicated that they were also responsible for witnessing the bodies of those who had died "before they bee [sic] suffered to bee buried."[8] In this statement, the use of the word "suffered" denoted an air of concern about the body being buried prior to being confirmed as being dead. After plague victims were confirmed as being dead, there was a short observational period when the body would receive last rites before being buried. According to the 1594 plague orders, all bodies of those who had died from the plague were to "be buried after Sunne [sic] setting, and yet neverthelesse [sic] by daylight."[9] Once it was confirmed and recorded that a person had died and been buried, their clothing and bedding were burned. If the loss of these items was greater than poor families could bear, a collection was taken up to compensate them for the loss.

Although the distributed plague orders included remedies which would allow people to provide treatments with easily affordable remedies, the end result was believed to be determined by God's will, including who survived. Despite this, people did their best to survive. To that end, remedies which appeared to have had positive effects during prior plague outbreaks were recycled whenever the plague reappeared. For instance, remedies that were initially issued by the Lord Mayor of London at the request of King Henry VIII were republished in the *Sundrie Approoved Remedies Against the Plague* sometime between 1584 and 1628. The goal of these remedies was to treat the symptoms of the plague, most notably to combat fever and remove the buboes. One remedy from *Sundrie Approoved Remedies Against the Plague* suggested that drinking a combination of rue, mandrake, oused, burnet, dragonroot, and featherfew would stop the plague from advancing if it was ingested after the fever presented but before the buboes appeared. The botanical reference guide *The Herball, or General Historie of Plantes* (1597) explained that each of these ingredients combatted a symptom of the plague or helped bring the remedy into the proper humoral balance. The plague remedies also included suggestions for preventative measures and to test lingering infection in a house. The tests differed by location and could be as simple as laying onions in a house and blowing on them with air from bellows or as cumbersome as farmers letting their sheep in the house for a few days, washing them, and feeding the dirty water to the pigs to see if the pigs would remain healthy.[10] The absorptive properties of onions were of particular interest. Onions would be used to test if plague had remained in a house and to remove the plague from a neighborhood. This was done by peeling a few onions and putting them on the ground for two weeks. When the onions changed color, it was assumed that it was because they had sucked up the disease and left the area free from plague.

One remedy from 1594 plague orders suggested that the air inside a room could be cleansed by submerging "a red-hot brick into a basin of vinegar."[11] In the play *The Alchemist* (1610), the character Face insisted that he was not infected by the plague, despite having recently visited a household that had been infected by the disease. When asked how he had escaped infection, he stated that he "burnt rose-vinegar, treacle, and tar" to sweeten the air so completely that no one would be able to tell that plague had been in the house.[12] These tests were not generally viable because evidence based medicine had not yet been developed to a science. Instead, the "evidence" that was valued came from testimonials of inhabitants who had not been reinfected. The casual mechanisms and reasons why a particular remedy worked were not considered to be as important and were studied with less zeal.

Despite the plague orders and the best attempts of the city administration of London to carry them out, London descended into complete chaos by the end of the summer of 1603. Overwhelmingly, the plague orders had been ignored by the citizens of London. People regularly attended public houses and taverns, went to work, and attended gatherings. Bedding and the personal effects of those who had died of the plague were thrown into the road, where they could not be avoided by those passing by. In an effort to regain control of the spread of the disease, all fairs and festivals within fifty miles of London were canceled. Any festivities that took place beyond the fifty mile radius denied admission to anyone who had been infected or had an infected person in their home since the beginning of July. Additionally, the city of London punished those who knowingly spread the disease or misinformation about it. People who ignored the quarantine orders could be flogged or sent to prison, depending on the severity of their transgression. Likewise, people who spread rumors about the infected being able to choose when they would die were "reprehended."[13] If the person spreading this misinformation was ecclesiastical, the Bishop of London added that they would be "forbidden to preache" and that they would be advised to "forbeare to beter [sic] such dangerous opinions upon paine of imprisonment."[14] The punishment would be enacted if they continued to spread misinformation. Despite these consequences, the death toll continued to rise to nearly 9,000 in August.

By the end of December 1603, just under 20 percent of the population of London (30,613) had died.[15, 16] In his *The Wonderful Yeare* (1603), the Elizabethan dramatist Thomas Dekker bemoaned the uselessness of the herbal remedies that so many depended on. He described the sound of tolling bells, as nature slowly reclaimed a city crying out in hollow desperation as the plague ravaged on:

> the bare ribbes of a father that begat him, lying there: here the Chaplesse hollow scull of a mother that bore him: round about him a thousand corses [sic], some standing bolt up right in their knotted winding sheetes: others half mouldred [sic] in rotten coffins, that should suddenly yawne wide open, filling his nosthails with noisome stench, and his eyes with the sight of nothing but crawling wormes.[17]

Gatherings and wakes to pay tribute to the dead had been forbidden, and the number of people who could attend the corpse to the grave was limited to six in August 1603. In his *The Seven Deadly Sinnes of London* (1606), Dekker wrote that these regulations were "cruel" and "barbarous" because they disrespected the dead and had such a great emotional toll on the living.[18] Addressing the city administration of London, he lamented, "Thou didst then take away all *Ceremonies* due unto them, and haldest [sic] them rudely to their last beds."[19] Plague pits were opened and bodies were pushed into them, protected only by their winding sheets. Of this Dekker described that the bodies were tumbled into "their everlasting lodgings (ten in one heape, and twenty in another) as if all the rooms upon earth had bin [sic] full."[20] Of that "noisome stench" Dekker warned that the foul smell of decay was poisonous. He warned against reopening graves and plague pits, even to add another body from the same household, for fear that the "rotten stenches, and contagious damps would strike up into thy nostrils."[21] Bodies that were buried in graveyards were done so in graves so shallow that body parts jutted out of the ground as it settled. The Anglican cleric, John Donne, compared these particular occurrences to the resurrection of Christ, in that "some of the dead arose out of their graves, that were buried again; so in this lamentable calamity, the dead were buried, and thrown up again before they were resolved to dust, and make room for more."[22] Donne went on to say that although these people had died, the part of them that God had breathed into them—the soul—was still alive and safe with God.

Theories of Contagion

London may have been affected by regular plague epidemics, but scientific study continued across Europe. As medical theory evolved towards the end of the seventeenth century and into the eighteenth century, medical scholars continued to theorize about the cause of disease. The physician Thomas Sydenham (1624–1689) and chemist Robert Boyle (1627–1691) developed a theory reminiscent of Paracelsus' astral poison. Rather than invisible emanations dropping from space, however, they theorized that epidemics were caused by particles that emanated "from the bowels of the earth [and] polluted the atmosphere."[23] Intertwined with the humoral theory, they believed that once the particles entered the atmosphere, they interacted with the air, the weather, and the humoral properties of the body. Sydenham theorized that any observational differences in symptoms during a disease outbreak were caused by how the atmospheric particles interacted with each person's humoral qualities. Prominent physicians praised this theory for its inclusion of the humoral theory, and it became the basis for much of the research on contagion during the beginning of the eighteenth century.

Despite Sydenham and Boyle's reliance on Hippocratic theories, other contagionist theorists chose to phase out the humoral factors. The first microscope had been invented during the early 1620s. It used the same technology as the telescope: mounting a concave lens and a convex lens on either side of a rigid tube to magnify objects that were too small to be seen by the naked eye. The German scholar Athanasius Kircher (1602–1680) studied pus and blood from plague patients, through the lens of this kind of microscope. Although this low-powered microscope would not have been strong enough to see the *yersinia pestis* bacteria, Kircher described seeing "countless broods of worms" in the blood.[24] He built on the theories of Fracastoro by identifying that people became sick after eating food that flies who had fed "on the juices of the diseased and dying" had landed on.[25] The existence of bacteria was identified in the 1670s by the Dutch scientist Antoni van Leeuwenhoek (1632–1723). Terming his new discovery "animalcules," Leeuwenhoek conducted experiments to find out where they came from, why they existed in a variety of sizes, why they behaved differently from each other and how they should be distinguished and classified.[26]

Plague outbreaks continued into the eighteenth century, and the medical community continued to study them. The English physician Richard Mead (1673–1754) studied the bubonic plague and published the resulting theories on disease transmission in his *Short Discourse Concerning Pestilential Contagion and the Method to Be Used to Prevent It* (1720). This Fellow of the Royal Society and the Royal College of Physicians instructed that the best way to keep from catching the plague was to stay away from contagions. It was still not understood that the bubonic plague was caused by rat fleas, so Mead surmised that disease was transmitted through the air, from "diseased persons," or via goods that originated from "infected places."[27] Other causes of infectious diseases included the bad smells wafting off of stagnated water, "putrid Exhalations from the Earth; and above all, the Corruption of dead *Carcasses* lying unburied."[28] He believed that while air could transport the disease, the initial contagion had to come from within a person. The transmission would be completed when a healthy person inhaled the infected particles, and they began to putrefy and ferment inside their body. He theorized that people themselves became spreaders of contagion as the particles fermented inside them and spread outward through their bodily functions.

As the eighteenth century proceeded, theories about contagion began to replace the competing theories regarding the harm that could be caused by bad air or how weather affected the body. Due to the inability for most people to see Kircher's "little worms" or Leeuwenhoek's "animalcules" the theoretical understanding of disease as something that occurred inside the body was slow to gain acceptance. Their theories gained in popularity during the nineteenth century, after the magnifying power of microscopes had strengthened enough to make bacteria easier to see and observe.

The Study of the Functionality of the Heart

Regarding the budding study of anatomy, physicians and scholars continued to investigate how the heart worked beyond what had been written by Galen and Vesalius. They attempted to answer questions about the blood's origin and what caused it to flow throughout the body. The ancient scholars had claimed that "the liver was the center of the blood system."[29] It was believed that once food was consumed it became a "natural spirit." These natural spirits were then absorbed by the liver, which in turn released blood that flowed throughout the body. Once the natural spirits left the liver, they moved through the body until they reached the brain and then flowed over the nerves in order to activate the body. Although the ancient scholars were aware of the existence of the heart, they misinterpreted its functionality. They believed that the heart and lungs worked together to maintain the blood's temperature, with the heart-warming the blood and the lungs cooling it.[30]

In 1606, the Italian physiologist Andrea Cesalpino (1524–1603) hypothesized that blood flowed from the heart through the pulmonary artery, aorta, vena cava, and the pulmonary vein.[31] In 1559, Realdo Colombo (1515–1559) published his research in *De re Anatomica*, where he explained his observations regarding the role of the veins and pulmonary arteries in pulmonary circulation. His work built on the theories of Vesalius and began to definitively disprove Galen's theory regarding how blood moved around the heart. Colombo's theory explained why blood could be found in the pulmonary veins, while simultaneously removing the necessity for interventricular septal pores for the blood to move through:

> Between these ventricles there is a septum through which almost everyone believes there opens a pathway for the blood from the right ventricle to the left, and that the blood is rendered thin so that this may be done more easily for the generation of vital spirits. But they are in great error, for the blood is carried through the pulmonary artery to the lung and is there attenuated; then it is carried, along with air, through the pulmonary vein to the left ventricle of the heart. Hitherto no one has noticed this or left it in writing, and it especially should be observed by all.[32]

These new findings were instrumental in evolving theories relating to the functionality of the heart and made way for William Harvey's work in the 1620s and 1630s.

Dr. William Harvey, followed in the footsteps of Paracelsus and Vesalius because he believed that empirical evidence was more valuable than the writings of the ancient scholars. He also built on the theories of Cesalpino and Colombo in his personal studies on the human heart and blood circulation. A leader in his field, he had attained the respect of his fellow physicians and King James I early in his career. After obtaining his medical degree at the University of Padua, he worked as faculty at the University of Cambridge for two years before moving to London. He became a Fellow at the College of Physicians in 1607 and two years later he was appointed as a physician to St. Bartholomew's Hospital, a position he earned with a distinguished recommendation from King James I, the president of the College, and the endorsement of the senior fellows. In 1618, he received an appointment to serve as the physician to King James I.

Even as he theorized about the anatomical functions of the human heart, Harvey was cognizant of the risk involved in challenging Galen. Despite the medical community's continued push away from the writings of the ancient scholars, their theories were still considered to be the cornerstone of medicine. Therefore, challenging them could come at a high price, like it had for Paracelsus. Harvey utilized his position at the RCP as a sounding board for his theories on circulation for nearly a decade before writing his *Anatomical Essay on the Motion of the Heart and Blood in Animals* (1628). By building on the anatomical and physiological theories of his predecessors, Harvey's experiments on blood circulation ushered in a new era of physiology. In his *Anatomical Essay...*, Harvey identified that "the blood circulates, revolves, propelled and then returning, from the heart to the extremities, from the extremities to the heart, and thus that it performs a kind of circular motion."[33] In the same book, he also explored the concept that life began and ended with the palpitations of the heart and stated that "the heart is the principle of life."[34]

In his *De Mortu Cordis* (1628) Harvey proved that the heart pumped blood and caused it to circulate throughout the body. In his opening letter of his book he explained to King Charles I that "the heart of animals is the foundation of their life, the sovereign of everything within them ... from which all power proceeds."[35] Similar to Galen's experiments, Harvey's initially experimented on sheep and pigs. He believed that since humans were animals, the theories governing their bodies would be similar. From these experiments, he was able to theorize that blood circulated around the body. His later experiments on humans showed that when a tourniquet was applied to an arm, it would cause "the veins to become engorged and that blood can only be milked from an engorged vein ... towards the heart—but when the vein is thus emptied it only fills from the periphery."[36] He also noticed that if the tourniquet was applied quickly and fastened tightly, the arm would lose its color and the veins would not engorge. Therefore, he concluded (1) that arteries transitioned blood to the veins and (2) that there were "capillary anastomoses between arteries and veins."[37] Unfortunately, the latter conclusion was not proven until after his death. With the acceptance of pulmonary circulation and systemic circulation, the medical community considered blood circulation to be a definitive sign of life by the eighteenth century. Likewise, having a better understanding the functionality of the heart led the medical community to conclude that the cessation of a heartbeat was a sign of death.

Although Harvey is most remembered for his research on the heart, he continued to study blood and published new theories on disease transmission and susceptibility. Focusing, in part, on diseases that were transferred to humans through animal bites, he observed that if a rabid dog bit a person, the bite location could heal, but the person could still become feverish and suffer the symptoms of rabies. He believed that the person was so affected because the blood transported the contagium to the heart, where it "kindled" the beginning of a fever, and both the contagium and the fever circulated it throughout the body. He also theorized that either a fever or medication that was taken internally had the power to destroy the contagium that was making the body sick. Meanwhile, medical remedies that were applied externally were "absorbed" into the body and into the bloodstream. Once the external medication had entered the blood, its positive effects were delivered to the part of the body that needed it in order to be effective.

Medical Practitioners and Practices

The medical community also faced the challenge of bridging the gap between academic medicine and the medicine used to treat the average person. During the two preceding centuries minerals (such as sulphur and mercury) and gemstones (such as rubies and emeralds) began to make their way into the medical pharmacopeia. The following recipe for face cream was developed in by the French physician Nostradamus (1503–1566); it was toxic due to the inclusion of mercury and lead. For the best outcome, this skin cream was supposed to be worn until it turned gray and then removed. It was used to remove blemishes of all types, leaving behind only the purest of skin.

> Take six ounces of mercuric chloride, put it in a clean marble mortar, pound it finely with a wooden pestle and continue doing so, though in a place out of the wind, for almost a whole day, until it is as fine as possible. You will then soon see that it is like finely ground flour and when you take it in your hand you will notice no course bits and it will run very gently through your fingers. Now stir in with it the spittle of a young man who, for three days, has neither eaten garlic, nor onions, or vinegar, nor anything disagreeable and, when you have stirred it for a good while, add pure mercury to it and strain it through a white, thick and well-cleaned woolen cloth Next take as much as six drachms (or as much as six shining crowns) of lead and tin and three grains of ground silver, mix these ingredients up continuing to add the spittle of a young man. Do this for as long as it takes for the mercury to appear really white, for when the mercury is first mixed with the mercuric chloride it turns black and soon afterwards grey.[38]

The expense of mercury and silver limited the use of this recipe to the rich. Such was the case for many new medical discoveries, and the medical community was split on how to handle this issue. Some believed that the newest discoveries should only be practiced on those who could afford them. There was a long held belief by the nobility of England and France, for example, that the touch of the king could cure ailments of all sorts. Of course, this was only available to those who ranked the highest in society. Meanwhile, other people believed that medicine and medical advancements should be made available to the average person. One of the most influential medical professionals who agreed with the latter sentiment was Nicholas Culpeper.

Nicholas Culpeper's story weaves through the undercurrent of the seventeenth century like English ivy climbs up the side of a house. He was born to the rector of the parish of Ockley (Surrey, England), the Reverend Nicholas and his wife Mary Culpeper, nee Attersoll, in 1616. Due to his father's untimely death that same year, Nicholas and his mother returned to her hometown of Isfield, Sussex, where her father, William Attersoll, served as the rector and guided the town with strict Puritan views. When Attersoll's daughter and grandson arrived at his home, he promptly stepped into the patriarchal role, tutoring young Nicholas in theology, the writings of the ancient scholars, astrology, and mathematics. He taught Nicholas with the same Puritanical rigidity with which he led his congregation. Soon, rumors began to circulate that Nicholas was difficult to control and did not act like the ideal obedient son.

During his childhood, Nicholas spent his time with his mother and the other women in the scullery. From them, he learned how to clean and prepare food and medicine. His mother was known for her ability to mix medicines and treat wounds using remedies that were shared and handed down from generation to generation. One of his chores was collecting the herbs necessary to both make these remedies and flavor the food being cooked. Although Hippocrates had thought that food was different than medicine and should be prepared as such, in seventeenth-century Isfield, the two were intrinsically blended. Through these experiences, Nicholas learned about herbs such as honeysuckle (used to treat sunburn) and clary (used to strengthen backs) and the importance of the different parts of bracken. Bracken is a short plant with fern like fronds that were "suffused with a form of cyanide."[39] However, the roots of bracken could be added to honeyed water or mead and applied to the itching caused by threadworm. Additionally, burning bracken leaves would repel gnats and other small bugs that would bite people as they slept on their straw filled mattresses.

In 1632, Nicholas attended Cambridge University to study liberal arts like his father (Culpeper) and grand-father (Attersoll). The liberal arts classes expanded his understanding of mathematics, grammar, and astronomy—which continued to work in conjunction with astrology. In addition, he was taught rhetoric, logic, music, and geometry. While studying at Cambridge, he was also introduced to the joy of smoking tobacco, an increasingly popular comfort.

During the preceding century, English merchants had bought their tobacco from Spain, until the two countries went to war in the latter part of the century. During the 1620s, tobacco began to be imported to England from the British colony of Virginia. As tobacco became more popular with the young, it was condemned by the older generation. A bill was passed by the House of Commons to ban it, although the ban was never enforced. Trusted authorities such as William Vaughan, the author of *Directions for Health* (1600), and King James I published literature condemning the vice of tobacco, claiming that it caused the senses to dull, the brain to slow, and infertility in both men and women. Despite the King's aversion to it, tobacco was found to have several medical uses. Tobacco leaves were turned into tea or sucked on so that the juices could soothe coughs or sore throats and acted as an expectorant for chest congestion. The smoke was said to dull the ache of headaches. When the plague returned to London in 1665, people smoked a mixture of tobacco, sulphur, and amber as a preventative measure. By the end of his reign, even King James I began to enjoy smoking tobacco.

Despite the purported healing effects of tobacco, medicine of the middle of the seventeenth century had generally evolved into more complex compounds than the herbal based remedies of the centuries before. In London, apothecaries were similar to modern pharmacies and were responsible for the creation of medicinal drugs. In a world filled with guilds and companies where similar trades could band together in order to gain political and social validity, the apothecaries were situated under the Grocer's Company because they sold derivatives of spices and edible products. Items sold to the public included mulled wines, herbs, and medicinal drugs that were created in-house. It was expected that apothecaries would be pious and clean, have a working knowledge of herbs, and have the necessary equipment create the medicines that were prescribed by physicians.

The College of Physicians took an interest in the apothecaries during the seventeenth century. They were concerned about regulating the drugs being dispensed. Unfortunately for them, the Society of Apothecaries (SoA) had set itself up to be self-regulating at its inception in 1617. It is important to note that those regulations were not assurances that the medicines were effective. Efficacy regulations were not put in place until the twentieth century, some as late as the 1960s. Instead, the SoA focused on regulating the training that apprentices received, ensuring that the medicines created were of high quality and punishing those who created false or fraud medicines.[40]

Much like the College of Physicians oversaw the practice of medicine in London, the Society of Apothecaries oversaw apothecary shops throughout the city. The standard apothecary apprenticeship lasted seven to eight years, during which time they would learn about botany and chemistry. Both of these subjects were considered to be very important when it came to understanding how to properly combine herbs into medicinal compounds. Apprentices became familiar with the different parts of plants, herbs, and fruits and were expected to understand their therapeutic properties well enough to combine them into different medicines, salves, boluses, teas, and pills. Practicing members were also responsible for maintaining the respectability of the shops by confiscating rotting goods and punishing those who engaged in malpractice.

* * *

Just after the London plague outbreak of 1625, Nicholas Culpeper left Cambridge for London. He became an apprentice at Simon White's apothecary shop. The shop was located at the Temple Bar, between the tightly packed houses of Fleet Street and the growing metropolis of Newgate Street, and was within walking distance to the Thames River, St. Paul's Cathedral, and St. Bartholomew's Hospital. The shop was perfectly positioned to greet sailors as they came in from their worldwide travels. It catered to those working in the businesses nearby. Marketing was exceptionally important to maintain interest in White's apothecary shop. New fruit or small treasures that were given as gifts or bartered for services rendered from those who sailed abroad were placed in window displays as enticements to passersby.

The bustling metropolis of London was very different than the opulence to which Culpeper had become accustomed at Cambridge. He found himself working as an unofficial apprentice in White's humble apothecary shop, which often wanted for money. He would have been perfectly positioned to watch the world go by, if the world of 1630s London was there to be watched. On the contrary, the practice of medicine in the city was contentious at best. Not only were the physicians, barber-surgeons, and apothecaries vying for the people's patronage, money, and academic credence, but there was an array of other types of practitioners practicing different disciplines of medicine within the city.

Astrologists continued to use the movement of the stars and planetary bodies to predict how and when diseases would affect the city and the people within it. Horoscopes had gained popularity during the Renaissance.

Using multiple calculations, astrologists would start at the exact minute of a person's birth and the exact alignment of the planets at that time. A complex series of charts were referenced in order to determine what planetary forces affected that person's character, as well as the twelve facets of their lives that affected them the most. Like the humors of the ancient texts, it was believed that the planets that controlled these facets also controlled different parts of the human body. For example, according to the Paracelsian philosopher and physician, Robert Fludd (1574–1637), Sagittarius was responsible for ailments of the hips and upper legs while Gemini affected the fingers, shoulders, and arms.[41]

The study of alchemy was more complex than the fable of turning straw into gold. Alchemical medicine blended the still evolving concepts of medicine, science, and chemistry into one boiling pot of understanding. Elixirs were created by distilling or fermenting the chemical elements of base liquids, such as wine or vinegar. Similar to astrologists, alchemists believed that there was a direct connection between the human body and the universe. However, alchemists had not gained the respect of the medical community. Despite the popularity of apprenticeships throughout different disciplines of the medical community, alchemists maintained a code of secrecy. They used encoded texts, allegory, and symbolism to keep their craft secret and separate from the other medical practitioners of the time.

During the mid-seventeenth century, the belief of witchcraft had pervaded mainstream society. People believed that witches were responsible for causing illnesses and regarded the practice of witchcraft with superstition and fear. The persecution of witches began at the behest of Pope Innocent VIII in 1484 and was carried out throughout Catholic Europe by the Spanish Inquisition. This persecution continued throughout the sixteenth and seventeenth centuries, finally tapering off in the nineteenth century. Sorcery, pacts with the devil, weather control, and mind control were all lumped under the heading of "witchcraft." Although witchcraft was a more esoteric understanding of medicine, it existed alongside the more predominant theories of medicine.

Domestic medicine, or home remedies, continued to be a mainstay of popular medicine. During the Renaissance through the Romantic eras, most people were not able to accumulate savings. Therefore, the costs associated with seeing a physician and buying medicine from the apothecary were often out of reach for the common person. Generally administered by the women of the house, home remedies were passed down through the generations or shared by friends. They were made from seasonal ingredients that could be easily obtained and recipes that could be followed using equipment found in the home. Women were expected to be able to splint broken bones, pull teeth, and care for all manner of ills, from getting worms and bugs out of ears and noses to alleviating the symptoms of those suffering from smallpox, ague, influenza, and other common ailments. Imposters and quack doctors were also actively practicing medicine throughout London and England at large. Although witches were thought to cause harm to the people around them, these fake practitioners were actively unconcerned about causing harm. Unlike the remedies that were made by apothecaries, which may have had questionable effectiveness, quack medicines were never intended to be effective and may have even prolonged the illness or problem. Any positive effects attributed to these medicines were purely incidental. Quack doctors sold their remedies solely for money and cared little about the effects that their substances had on the patient.

In this sort of medical atmosphere, it was easy for the boundaries between each type of medical practice to become blurred. Although the different professional societies and guilds tried to work alongside each other, animosity arose when it was perceived that one organization was intruding on the scope of another. It became clear that the practice of medicine needed to be regulated throughout London. In order to do so, censors were deployed by the RCP to oversee the practice of medicine throughout the city. These censors were granted the authority to search, fine, press charges against, and punish those who practiced medicine outside the confines of the law. They were hypercritical of apothecary shops, which they lumped in with the less reputable factions of medicine, and would show up, unannounced, demanding to see paperwork, storerooms, and private areas, convinced that they would find illicit activity.[42]

Although most apothecaries were above board, there was reason for concern in the other areas of less reputable medical practice. Arthur Dee, the son of Queen Elizabeth I's advisor John Dee, for example was charged with being an impostor. He was ordered to bring his remedies before the censors so that a penalty could be imposed upon him. Similarly, John Lambe, the ex-protégé of the Duke of Buckingham was summoned before the censors for posing as a physician and selling medicine which he knew would not be effective. Not only did he sell false cures, but he did so for the tidy sum of £40–£50 each. This would have equated the 2020 purchasing power of approximately £8,395–£10,490, respectively.[43]

The concerns held by the Fellows of the College of Physicians were not without reason. Experience had taught them that when the lines between medical practices blurred, people died. Such was the case with the death of the prosperous London lawyer Joseph Lane. In April 1632, Lane had developed a recurring stomach issue. He sent his legal apprentice, Robert Cromwell, a cousin of the more famous Oliver Cromwell, to Christopher Matthews' apothecary shop for a purgative that had been previously prescribed by Lane's recently deceased physician. As requested, Matthews created the purgative potion. Initially, the potion seemed to work. However, when Lane's vomiting did not cease, he called upon the physician, Dr. Gifford, for assistance.

Upon observing Lane's symptoms of repeated vomiting and blackened mouth and gums, Gifford wrote out a different prescription. This one was for a large chewable pill, called a bolus, made of laudanum. The intent of using this opium-based drug was to settle the digestive system. Cromwell was sent back to Matthews' shop and returned shortly with the requested bolus. However, he was stopped by Lane's father-in-law, Dr. Francis Banister, who had arrived to take care of Lane during his illness. When Banister saw the bolus, he considered it to be suspect. Not only was it larger than it should have been, but it did not taste as it should have. Rather than giving it to Lane, he sent Cromwell back to the apothecary shop and requested that the bolus be remade. After spending the night with Lane, he noticed some very peculiar symptoms, such as bloody evacuations, convulsions and twisting of the body, as well as blackened gums, inflamed mouth, and smelly breath. He called for Dr. Gifford and discussed his suspicion that Lane was suffering from mercury poisoning. Lane died shortly after.[44]

The inquest into Joseph Lane's death occurred quickly. First, his apprentice, Cromwell, was arrested after it was discovered that he had purchased mercury sublimate at another apothecary shop. A similar white powder was identified in the initial bolus, which Banister had retained when he asked Cromwell to acquire a new one. Ultimately, Cromwell was imprisoned and hung on the charge of poisoning Joseph Lane.[45] The following month, King Charles II took an interest in this case. He asked that the College of Physicians perform their own investigation. Lane's body was exhumed, and two Fellows of the College performed an autopsy in front of "two other physicians and four surgeons."[46] Although they found signs of "inflammation and mortification in the body," the findings did not support the accusation of poisoning of any sort, including mercury.[47] These results were presented to the King by the President of the College on June 1, 1632.

These findings caused the College to take action against the apothecaries. They called for tighter restrictions and William Harvey took their requests to the Privy Council, who were responsible for advising the King. Primarily, the College wanted to disallow apothecaries from stocking the following poisonous items: refined mercury (precipitate and sublimate), opium, arsenic, orpiment, hellebore, colocynth (derived from the bitter apple plant), and a derivative of a Middle Eastern bindweed called scammony.[48] Additionally, the RCP requested a "Royal Edict under the most severe penalties, that no Apothecary for the future shall dare to compound for the Well, or administer to the Sick any medicines, especially Vomits, Purges, Opiates, Mercurial or Antimonial remedies without the prescription of Physicians then living," *and* they would have to produce the physicians receipt "upon the command or request of the Censors of the College."[49] If the apothecaries did not follow this order, or were unable to produce the doctor's receipt, the apothecary would be charged and legally punished "as a publick [*sic*] enemy to the life of man."[50] Finally, the RCP wanted the apothecaries to take an oath swearing that they would no longer create their own concoctions and would only use those set forth in the *Pharmacopeia Londinensis* (1618): the standardized list of medicines and ingredients that were used in England.

The Society of Apothecaries was not pleased and launched their rebuttal directly at Harvey, rather than at the College. They stated that the RCP did not know enough about how those ingredients should be used to make such demands. They cited a case where the apothecary for St. Bartholomew's created a medication at the behest of William Harvey. The core ingredient of this medicine was colocynth, which was such a powerful purgative that it caused both stool and fluid to evacuate through the bowels.[51] Due to its powerful purgative effects, this ingredient was only used in very small quantities of about five grains per concoction. It was the SoA's stance that Harvey requested that a drachm—roughly 12 times the recommended dosage—of colocynth be mixed with several ounces of wine. This overdose proved to be deadly to the patient who ingested it.

Harvey was not concerned about the accusation, most likely due to his Royal appointment by King Charles II. However, the apothecary's refusal to conform to the requests of the College caused much internal discussion. Over the winter of 1633–34, the College of Physicians debated how to keep the apothecaries compliant. As they discussed ideas, they shared stories about the disrespect that they had received from apothecaries. In response, they decided to invite the Society of Apothecaries to discuss overall situation and that the discussion should be led by William Harvey. On July 4, 1634, Harvey addressed the Society of Apothecaries. He told them that it was time that they took their business seriously. He encouraged them to conform in showing honesty and integrity when it came to their craft and to remember to keep their prices affordable. His condescending tone was not received well. Negative attitudes turned to anxiety when they were told that the College had requested that the Privy Council look into the Society's affairs.

Additionally, the College had used Harvey's royal connections to gain an audience in the Court of the Star Chamber to discuss their grievances with the SoA. The Court of the Star Chamber had been initially created to see cases that included powerful people who could intimidate a panel of jurors. It was held at Westminster Palace and grievances were told directly to Privy Counsellors. When the time for the trial came, over thirty apothecaries and apprentices were called into the Star Chamber. In their defense, the apothecaries aired their own grievances against the College. They thought that physicians, who were not familiar with the art of making medicines, were not qualified to search apothecary shops and test their products.[52] They also pointed out that the College had no business stating that they must adhere strictly to the *Pharmacopeia Londinensis* when the physicians prescribed medication that was not listed within it. Finally, they were resentful that the College of Physicians were able to examine its own apprentices, and the SoA was not granted the same ability.

The apothecaries also made a case to prove that their role in the medical community was just as important as the physicians. In addition to showcasing thriving apothecary shops, they brought forward the physician to the Czar of Russia, Arthur Dee, to speak on the behalf of the apothecaries. The same Arthur Dee who had been called out for his unscrupulous practices had attained his medical degree at the University of Basle and went on to a royal appointment. He had returned to London shortly before being asked to speak to the Star Chamber on behalf of the apothecaries. The statement that Dee delivered was complimentary of the apothecaries. The RCP and the SoA went back and forth with their accusations for so long that there did not seem to be a resolution.[53] This situation did not help smooth relations between the two professional associations.

As the validity of the Society of Apothecaries improved, it unnerved the College of Physicians, who wanted to hold their monopoly on supplying the more prestigious medical care in London. While both groups worked to bring better a better quality of health care to the citizens of London, they had to be cognizant of where the line separating their respective areas of expertise lay. Generally, the physicians who practiced under the RCP were responsible for providing medical care, while the apothecaries who practiced under the SoA were responsible for prescribing and dispensing medicine. There was also a difference between the communities that they serviced; the physicians tended to serve the wealthy classes, while the apothecaries primarily served the merchant and poor classes.

The line between the two blurred throughout the seventeenth century and culminated in a lawsuit between the two in 1701, when the apothecary, William Rose, visited a patient. The College of Physicians pressed charges against him that year for practicing medicine without holding their license. As the facts of the case were determined, it was discovered that Rose had been sent for by the patient, John Seale. Rose had delivered several medical remedies, such as "Bolus's, Electuaries, and Juleps," to Seale for a month before the College brought any charges against him.[54] Upon review by the jury and judges, it was determined that Rose's actions did not constitute "practicing physic," as intended by the Act of Parliament. Therefore, they ruled in favor of the apothecaries. Their ruling clarified the way that medicine was regulated in England. By giving the apothecaries the right to give medical advice as well as sell their medicines, they were effectively allowed to practice medicine. This, in turn, took the regulation of medicine in London away from the College and their censors. After the case, the regulatory authority of the censors decreased until their primary function was to arbitrate fees.[55]

After the 1634 case, apothecaries ceased giving physicians even the slightest bit of deferential treatment. It was in this political atmosphere that Nicholas Culpeper was presented to the Society of Apothecaries as an official apprentice. As part of his tenure being indentured to Simon White, he agreed to focus his time and efforts on the study of apothecary. He would live in White's home, follow his direction, pay for his own room and board, and keep away from romantic entanglements.[56] After seven years, he would be permitted to open his own shop. But that time was never going to come. In 1636, only two years into their formalized relationship, White's shop went bankrupt. Rather than remaining in London and opening another shop, White took the money that Culpeper had paid him for his apprenticeship and left for Ireland. Culpeper was left behind and found himself, once again, homeless, penniless, and alone.

The following year, the Society of Apothecaries set Culpeper up in a new apprenticeship with Francis Drake. Drake had a prosperous apothecary shop on Threadneedle Street in the Cornhill section of London. Misfortune visited again when Drake died in 1639. Once again, the SoA stepped in and placed Culpeper with a new master apothecary. This time he was apprenticed to Stephen Higgins, a founding member of the Society, who was nearing the end of his career. After realizing that he was paying for knowledge that was not being passed on to him, Culpeper decided to walk away from the apprenticeship system, leaving his education incomplete.

After stepping away from his training, Culpeper married Alice Field, who came from a wealthy family, and the two settled in northeast London near St. Mary's Spital, modernly known as Spitalfields. While there, he became reacquainted with Drake's former apprentice Samuel Leadbetter. Leadbetter agreed to unofficially apprentice Culpeper. They created and signed official apprenticeship papers that could be presented to the College or the censors if required. However, they did not consider it to be a legally binding agreement, and Leadbetter did not mentor Culpeper. Instead, Culpeper worked alongside Leadbetter, creating medicines and seeing patients.[57]

During this time Culpeper decided that he wanted to see patients, no matter how much—or how little—money they had. He decided to focus his practice on the common person, the poor, and the indigent. Overcrowding had long since been a problem in London, and landlords had broken up flats into tiny rent-a-rooms in order to pack in more people and earn more money from them. Public charities were no longer able to financially support the poor. On top of that, London's medical community was strained and poised to break apart. Respected institutions, such as St. Bartholomew's, had realized that they were seeing more poor patients than they could fiscally support.[58]

Recognizing the problem, Culpeper wanted to help fix it. He noticed that sometimes his patients were heartsick and sorrowful. This made sense since the average lifespan was only 32 years of age and over 25 percent of children did not live to see their fifteenth birthday.[59] Drawing upon his upbringing, he was able to provide them a little pastoral comfort. He promoted education, good hygiene, and healthy eating.[60] He viewed the body, mind, and soul as parts of the whole that worked in concert, all needing to be tended to in order for the person to truly heal.

When faced with ailments that required medical intervention, Culpeper insisted on using local ingredients that were prepared by simple processes. He strayed away from the poisons that had created such consternation between the College of Physicians and the Society of Apothecaries during the early 1630s. Opium, scammony and colocynths were not only hard for the body to process, but they were expensive ingredients. He understood that the chemicals and poisons included in the medical pharmacopeia could be used at certain times by people in better health. However, they were less helpful for the poorer, sicker clientele that he catered to. Using those types of ingredients would cause a drain on the bodies of people who were already suffering from malnourishment, fatigue, and a variety of other ills. Instead of making the medicine the focal point, he focused on the patient.

In addition to seeing patients, Culpeper began writing his own books on medicine. Most recognized for his *The English Physitian* (1652), Culpeper wrote on several topics including midwifery, astrology, and politics. He also translated the *Pharmacopeia Londinensis* into English in 1649. The College was none too pleased. Not only did his translation of the book make it accessible to more people, including those who were not traditionally educated, but he also added his own sections, including over 100 other plants that were not in the original source.[61]

One of his books, published three years after his death "laid down The Way and manner of finding out the Cause, Change, and End of the disease. Also whether the Sick be likely to live or die; and the Time when

2. Anatomy and Physiology in the Seventeenth Century   47

a Recovery or Death is to be expected. With the signs of Life or Death by the body of the Sick party; according to the judgement of Hippocrates."[62] In this book, Culpeper identified a problem that would take over the imaginations of physicians well into the nineteenth century. Up until this time, a cohesive definition of death had not been delineated. Death simply seemed to be the opposite of life; if a person was not living then they were dead. William Harvey had explored this issue in his *On the Motion of the Heart and Blood in Animals* (1628). In order to support his theory that the heart was the "principle of life," he described death as "a corruption which takes place through a deficiency of heat" and pointed out that "all living things are warm, [and] all dying things cold."[63] Culpeper focused his studies on the cause of death and how or when it evolved from life if the person was dying, or back to life when a person appeared to have already died. The answers to these questions were so mysterious that Culpeper turned to astrology to try to answer them. He believed that the planets and their astrological houses directly related to the recovery of a patient and whether that person was going to recover or die.

Despite how the theories of Nicholas Culpeper may fall on modern sensibilities, they were not without reason. The line between life and death was often blurred, especially without a cohesive definition of death. The lack of such a definition left the average person without any definitive understanding of the signs and symptoms of death and which of them were more certain than others. Things became even more complicated if the body was hastily buried because sometimes the perceived dead did not actually stay dead.

One such situation occurred in Kent, England, with a maid named Joan Bridges. On Sunday, August 16, 1646, Joan decided to skip church and spend the day with her friends at a local ale house. After imbibing heavily, she went home, where her siblings advised her to sleep off the effects of the alcohol. The next day, however, they found that they could not wake her. Her sister thought that Joan was in a trance, the catch-all name for a sleep disorder where the person could not be awakened. After trying to wake her, the sister declared her to be dead. The following day, Joan was laid into her coffin. Approximately 24 hours after it was believed that she had initially fallen into the trance, Jane was buried in the Rochester churchyard.

The next night, a man passing through the churchyard saw two dogs scratching and digging at Joan's grave. He heard a noise coming from the grave but walked on after it stopped. Upon hearing the noise again, he went to people who lived nearby to let them know that Joan Bridges had been buried alive. Despite her siblings' disinterest at the news, the townswomen gathered funds to exhume the body. When the coffin was opened, they found evidence that Joan had been prematurely buried. The cloth that had been tied around her face was taken off, and her nose and cheeks were "beaten flat."[64] The string that had tied "her toes together had torn the skin from the bone."[65] Her hands ripped "open her very bowels; her left hand sticking in her belly, and her right hand having razed [sic] the skin and flesh from her side."[66] Rumors started to circulate claiming that Joan's body still had some warmth in it when she had been laid to rest. Others claimed that her siblings' disinterest in the possibility of Joan being buried alive indicated that they had something to gain from her death. Still others thought that Joan had been beaten prior to being buried. However, those who saw the body exhumed refuted this claim because they felt that the damage occurred post-burial.

Similar stories were reported throughout England and Europe between the seventeenth and nineteenth centuries. These stories included themes of near misses, wherein people had been diagnosed as dead but recovered their senses prior to being closed into their coffin or committed to the grave. Other stories emerged about people awakening while resurrectionists were trying to steal their bodies or grave-robbers were trying to steal valuables out of their graves or tombs.

Although it is reasonable to assume that most premature burials did not occur with bad intentions, sometimes they did. A story befitting that of the loathsome Thénardiers' from Victor Hugo's *Les Misérables* (1862) was published in an anonymously written pamphlet from 1661. Laurence Cawthorn was a butcher who lived in the St. Nicholas Shambles section of Newgate Market, London (today at the corner of King Edward Street and Newgate Street). He was a young, healthy man who had recently completed his apprenticeship and took up lodging in a public house owned by William Cook.

After a hard day of work, and an evening of hard drinking, Cawthron returned to his rooms. He requested to be awoken at 3 a.m. in order to give himself time to kill and prepare the meat that he was planning on selling at the market. But when the landlord knocked to wake him that morning, he did not rise. Even as the morning drew on and the other butchers started to fill the market, Cawthorn did not rise. The landlord returned to his door, knocking and calling in an attempt to wake him up, but Cawthorn did not stir. As Cook became more curious about what had happened, he attempted to open the door but was unable to do so. After retreating back downstairs and discussing the matter with his wife and others, they decided to break open the door.

Upon gaining entrance to the room, they found Cawthorn "lying all along much like a dead man."[67] Despite this claim, witnesses in the room attested that he blinked a few times when his name was called. Others said that while they did not see him blink, they rubbed his arms to wake him and noticed that his body was warm. Despite this, "the Master of the house and his wife pull[ed] off his cloathes [*sic*], and fairly lay him in the bed."[68] As the group assembled discussed what to do next, it was disclosed that Cawthorn sometimes had "strange fits," where he would "lie in a trance like a dead man for many hours together."[69]

By the time the market was about to open for the morning, the decision was made that Cawthorn was dead and the searchers were called for. Upon review of the body, it was determined that he had died of quinsy, which causes the throat to swell and can slowly suffocate a person by restricting their airflow. The landlord's wife was ready to bury him that night. But others considered the action to be suspicious and voiced concerns about her intentions; was she trying to bury him quickly so that she could take possession of his belongings? Instead, she went around to the owners of other public houses and requested that they help pay for the burial. She claimed that his rent was so far in arrears that she and her husband could not possibly make up the debt on their own. However, her lust for money was well known, as was the fact that she would not let Cawthorn continue to live there if he was so far behind in his rent. Unable to obtain monetary assistance and despite the neighbor's nattering, she prepared Cawthorn for burial.

Although there were some reports that witnesses saw the body move as it was being carried to the gravesite, the burial went on as planned. The following day, Laurence Cawthorn was buried in a shallow grave in the common area of the Christ Church Blackfriars cemetery. That weekend people heard groans and shrieks coming from the gravesite, causing them to exhume the body three days later. Upon being removed from the grave, people noticed that Cawthorn had torn open his burial shroud and that his "eyes were swollen, and the brains beaten out of the head."[70] The landlord and his wife were brought before a jury and the Lord Mayor intended to bring them up on charges for their decision to hastily bury the young man. Unfortunately, the archival record runs dry and whatever happened to Mr. and Mrs. Cook has been lost to history.

CHAPTER 3

The Body, the Soul,
and the Diagnosis of Death

An attendant of a Princess suffered from "a violent nervous disorder."[1] One day, her lips paled, and her body temperature dropped. Those around her believed that she had died, and she was placed in her coffin. On the day of her funeral, just as the lid was about to be nailed onto her coffin, she revived. After her recovery, she said that she had been "perfectly conscious of all that happened around her."[2] She had heard what her friends said as they stood beside her coffin and lamented about her death. She felt herself be dressed in her burial clothes and be laid into her coffin, at which point, she had been struck with a feeling of anxiety. "She tried to cry out, but her soul was without power, and she could not act on her body."[3] It made her feel as though she was simultaneously inside and outside of her body.

* * *

Beginning in the Middle Ages people started to worry about preparing the soul before death. If a person died by causes that were not disease or age related, it was considered to be an unnatural death. Common causes of unnatural deaths included deadly accidents, homicide, dying in battle, or anything that did not give the person time to adequately prepare their soul for the journey to the afterlife. Since life was full of uncertainties, the church encouraged people to care for their souls while they were alive so that they would be in a state of perpetual readiness for the inevitability of death. People worked hard during their lifetimes both to survive and to fulfill their end of the promise that hard work in the mortal realm would result in better treatment once the body and the soul reconnected during the Reckoning. Simply contemplating death was an important part of the preparation. Other parts of the process included avoiding sins and "making spiritual reparation through contrition and penance" when sins could not be avoided.[4] To buy people some time to prepare, symptoms such as the shaking of the hands, inability to speak, loss of hearing, lowered body temperature, and a rattling cough were identified as signs of impending death. It was hoped that identifying the signs of approaching death would give the dying person enough time to properly prepare the soul before their demise.

What happened to the soul after the death of the body has been of particular interest historically. The concept of purgatory as a place where the sinful soul could repent and become fit for entry into Heaven was formalized during the Middle Ages. The belief that the prayers of the living could lessen the suffering of the purgatory-trapped soul helped this theory become widely accepted by Catholics by the fourteenth century.[5] It remained a universal Christian belief until the late seventeenth century and retained its importance even longer for Roman Catholics.

Theological conundrums began to occur during the Middle Ages when people regained consciousness after they had already been proclaimed as dead. In some cases, revival from apparent death was considered to be a miracle. When these incidents were noticed, sometimes questions were raised about why the consciousness had returned to the body and what it meant for the soul. Questions of this nature were considered to be so important in fifteenth-century England that they were sometimes directed to King Henry VI (1421–1471) to try to answer. During his reign, King Henry VI was known as a God-fearing and simple man who did not have "a crook or craft or untruth" within him.[6] He devoted more of his efforts to religious scholarship than to governing his country. Despite his poor leadership qualities, he was well-known and respected for his piety. After his death, he became the focal point of a cult who revered him and sought to canonize him. His reputation for being pious and virtuous worked in his favor, and a list of over 170 miracles were credited to him at the turn of the following century. Several of those miracles included the resurrection of children who appeared to be dead due to drowning. In one alleged miracle, a child had sunk to the bottom of a pond and remained there for over an hour before being revived.[7] Although he was not canonized, the debates about his deeds raised questions about the connection between the soul and a person's consciousness. People researched and debated how interrelated the two were and if one was responsible for the other. These questions were not answered during the Middle Ages, and theological debates on the subject continued for centuries.

The concept of the soul has been discussed since ancient Greece, when it was believed that the soul was an immortal being that was created by the Gods and was deposited into the body upon conception. By the Middle Ages, Christians believed that the soul could be destroyed. The destruction of the soul was considered to be a sign of death, so knowing where it was located and how it influenced the body was important. Several scholars in the Church of England followed the early Christian writings of the second-century African scholar, Tertullian (155–220 CE), who wrote "that the soul was material," meaning that it was physical and, therefore, could be destroyed.[8] By the Renaissance, the Catholic ecclesiastical councils had come to the conclusion that the soul was immortal and slept in the dead body until Judgment Day, at which time it would be absorbed back into the universe.[9] The most common seventeenth-century belief about what happened to the body and soul after death was called Christian moralism, which theorized that "the whole individual died and was insensible until the resurrection and judgment, at which time the whole individual would be resuscitated and enter on eternal life."[10] This theory stood in direct contrast with the Anglican view, of the early sixteenth century, which theorized that "the soul would go to heaven or hell immediately on death."[11] Searching for scientific answers to religious mysteries denoted a clear detachment from the blind faith in Christian doctrine and foreshadowed the scientific reasoning that termed the eighteenth century "the Enlightenment."

Debates relating to what material constituted the soul and how it worked in conjunction with the body continued throughout the seventeenth century. As the functionality of human anatomy continued to be studied, theories regarding how the mind interacted with the soul and/ or the body were incorporated into the debate. It was during this time that the naturalist René Descartes (1596–1650) conducted various studies on animal life, including human life. Like Paracelsus, he believed that humans were part of nature; therefore, his theories included how humans were affected by nature. After conducting numerous autopsies on both animals and humans, Descartes reported that he had never observed material within the body that could be considered a soul. Therefore, he concluded that it was not located within the torso or extremities of the body. In his *Treatise of Man* (written around 1633, published posthumously in 1662), Descartes conceptualized how the body and the soul were interrelated. He wrote about a type of man who had been created by God and was comprised of only the body and the soul. In this conceptualized model, the body was an earthen-made machine. Using mechanical instructions, he discussed different anatomical and physiological functions of the body including what made the heart-beat, how food was digested, how the body slept and awoke from a sleeping state, and how it sensed, internalized, and remembered external stimuli such as light, sound, tastes, smells, and temperature.[12]

Academic philosophy had previously attributed functions such as digestion and the ability to see, hear, taste, smell, and the regulation of body temperature to the soul and its command over the body. Descartes disagreed with that theory. He concluded that the body needed blood and "animal spirits" to be agitated by the heat of the heart in order to be able to move and live.[13] Since he had not been able to find these spirits residing in any other area of the body, he theorized that the soul and animal spirits were located inside the pineal gland at the center of the brain. He believed that thoughts originated in the central cavity and that the animal spirits inside received sensory information from the body, which they then imprinted onto the pineal gland, allowing for them to be perceived by the soul. In response, the soul, animal spirits, or a strong sensory response would then cause the body to move.

Inspired by the works of Descartes, the Italian physician Giovanni Lancisi's (1654–1720) book on the medical problem of sudden death, *De Subitaneis Mortibus* (1707), also touched briefly on the duality of the body and soul in human physiology. Lancisi defined life as "the organic structure of the solid parts of a major function, and at the same time to corresponding mixture, to the fluidity and mass of liquid parts of like function."[14] To Lancisi, the soul's influence was one of rational control over the body. Similarly, he theorized that death was caused by an obstruction or a defect within the system. He disagreed with Descartes' assertion that the soul was located near the center of the brain. Instead, Lancisi believed that it was located in the thick nerve bundle that connects the two hemispheres of the human brain: the corpus callosum. He asserted that sensations were brought to the corpus callosum and the thoughts that guided bodily movements were generated from there.[15] He supported the theory of the active or thinking soul and believed that it left the body as a person died.

Nicholas Culpeper had placed a high value on the importance on caring for the mind and the soul when the body was unwell. Lancisi echoed this sentiment but not in a way that may be expected. Sudden deaths were considered to be more dire than gradual deaths because they did not allow time for repentance or confession. This meant that person's soul was not properly prepared for the afterlife. Lancisi believed that it was the doctor's responsibility to gain the patient enough time for a priest to administer the appropriate Catholic sacraments prior to the person's death. Doing so was necessary in order "to avoid putting souls and the social order at risk by death without penitence and the opportunity to write a last will and testament."[16] If a person died without repenting and feeling contrite for their sins, they risked not being forgiven for those sins and being denied entrance into Heaven. According to Lancisi, the best ways to prepare the soul for death were to perform acts of penitence and contrition during daily life, or to hope for divine intervention.[17]

Scholars also debated what precisely happened when a person regained consciousness after they had already been diagnosed as dead. Since the person had been able to come back to life, it was generally assumed that the soul had not completely diminished or left the body. People often turned to the Bible in order to understand why this had happened. A popular reference relating to misdiagnosed death during the seventeenth and eighteenth centuries was the story of Lazarus of Bethany, in the Gospel of John. The Bible indicated that all men are supposed to die *once*. Making sure that it only happened once was the goal of the medical and religious communities during the eighteenth century. When people were misdiagnosed as dead, they were pre-empting this allowance. Coming back to life after they were proclaimed to be dead, and especially after the funeral, gave the appearance that the person had lived and died twice.

In the story of Lazarus of Bethany, Jesus' friend Lazarus died after an illness. Upon hearing that his friend was sick, Jesus decided to visit him. Before leaving, Jesus told his disciples that Lazarus was sleeping and that he was going to wake him up. Upon arriving in Bethany and being informed that Lazarus had died, Jesus assured the family that Lazarus would "rise again."[18] The Rev. Donald J. Bretherton of Canterbury surmised that Jesus was not referring to the "resurrection of the faithful," where the body would rise during the "Last Day."[19] Instead, the Reverend Bretherton explained that Jesus was referring to a much more immediate revival of Lazarus' body. Upon going to Lazarus' tomb, Jesus was met with resistance when he requested that it be opened. People were uninterested in seeing or smelling a rotting corpse. However, he persisted, and the tomb was opened. After praying at the tomb, Jesus summoned Lazarus to come out, surprising many when Lazarus did so under his own power.

There has been some debate about Jesus' meaning when he told the disciples that Lazarus was asleep. According to the Reverend Bretherton, the word for sleep (*katheudō*) was sometimes used to imply "physical death" in the New Testament, and other times it was used to identify a period of "natural sleep."[20] However, when Jesus referred to Lazarus, he used the word *koimaomai*. Since both of these words were used when Jesus woke the disciples out of their slumber in Gethsemane (Luke 22:45), it is feasible that Jesus thought that Lazarus was sleeping and that he would be able to assist in his friend's recovery.[21] However, according to Leon Morris, in his *The Gospel According to St. John* (1971), the verb that was used to imply that Lazarus was sleeping was supposed to mean "where the continuing state is meant."[22] In this case, "continuing" meant permanent or irreversible. Bretherton pointed out that if Morris' translation was applied, then it would leave room for the body to be apparently dead and resuscitated back to life, instead of actually being dead. This would allow the consciousness to return to the body and would give Lazarus the appearance of coming back from the dead. Likewise, there has been debate about Lazarus' actual state of death. Generally, the story focuses on the miracle of Jesus bringing him back from actual death to physical life. John Marsh pointed out that this conceptualization of the story struck a similar chord to that of Jesus causing the blind to be able to see. However, Marsh emphasized that the miracle was not in bringing Lazarus back to life. Rather, that it was that "a man, dead or alive, hears the voice of the Son of God and lives."[23] But since an actually dead person cannot hear, it has been postulated that Lazarus was not actually dead to begin with and had already been restored to life. This restoration was alluded to by John (the disciple) because he made no mention of the stench of decay after Lazarus' tomb had been opened. Bretherton also noted that when Jesus called for Lazarus to come out of his tomb, the wording used (*ho tethnēkōs*) indicated "a continuing condition, rather than the absolute finality of death."[24] Therefore, it was more likely that Lazarus' condition had remained in a stable state, rather than transitioning from death to life.[25] In addition to these theological debates, the believability of the story is also important. In this case, the importance stands with the fact that it was believed that someone (who was not the Son of God) could have appeared to die and then returned to life.

The proclamation that someone who had died returned to life was also made regarding the Lutheran prophet, John (Hans) Engelbrecht of Brunswick (1599–1642). Born at the cusp of the seventeenth century, Engelbrecht's story was published in a book titled *The German Lazarus*, which was translated into English in 1707. In 1622, Engelbrecht choked on a morsel of fried fish and panicked. He feared that he would not be able to receive his final sacrament before dying. As death drew near, he felt as though the devil was tormenting him, making him feel despondent, and causing him pain. He felt as though "a great many Knives had been struck into [his body]."[26]

It was reported that he cast out the devil with prayer and over the span of about twelve hours he felt himself slowly slip into death. He felt his body grow stiff and his limbs become cold. He lost each of his senses in turn, first his sight, then his ability to taste, and, finally, his hearing. He reported feeling as though he was being carried away before conversing with an unidentified presence. First, he was brought to the gates of Hell, where he saw the most intimidating darkness and heard the screams of the souls tortured within it. Again he prayed, this time through his spirit, and the Hellish presence before him disappeared. In its place the Holy Ghost appeared "in the shape of a white Man, who after having plac'd [*sic*] me on a Golden Chariot, carried me up into the glorious Light of the Divine

Brightness."[27] Upon being admitted into Heaven, he saw a choir of "spiritualized" prophets, apostles, and "Holy Angels" singing comforting music in "Heavenly Tongues."[28] One of the Holy Angels let him know that Jesus wanted him to return to earth and let others know what he had seen of both Heaven and Hell, after which he was returned to his body. His experience made him realize that the soul was actively integrated with his body. He described the integration as his body acting "like a dead *Glove*," unable to move without "a living hand" inside of it.[29] In this way, he described that the soul acted as the life force of a person and was responsible for controlling the movement of the body.

The Medical Narrative and Identifying Death

As the religious communities worked to identify the corporeal location of the soul, the medical community worked to identify a clinical definition of death. The separation of the soul from the body was one of the leading signs of death. Others included the cessation of automatic functions, the cessation of movement, and the loss of awareness or consciousness. Building off of the research of Descartes and Lancisi, the medical, scientific, and religious communities developed their theories in tandem as they attempted to properly and regularly identify the signs of death in order to save lives and to save souls. The German physician Christian Garmann (1640–1708) wrote that corpses remained semi-sentient. He believed that the corpse had the ability to hear and to feel pain even after life had been completely extinguished from the body. He pointed out that although a dead body moved differently than a living body, it still continued to move.[30] Relying on stories from the time of Pliny through the seventeenth century, Garmann noticed a trend where people implored those who dealt with corpses to be kind and gentle to them, lest they have bad memories of their own deaths.

Historically, the over-arching goal of the advancement of medical theory has been to keep people alive. This was also true during the eighteenth century. The prominent physicians in London were especially interested in gaining a better understanding of anatomy, physiology, and understanding the mystery of death. An article in the April 2, 1741, edition of the *Stamford Mercury* reported that "the Right Hon. The Earl of Waldegrave, who had been given over by his Physicians (which occasion'd the Report of his being dead) is now said to be a little better."[31] Misunderstandings such as this occurred due to the budding tests for death and because of the ambiguous definition of death. Beyond the medical concepts of the apparent and absolute stages of death, there was a profound lack of basic understanding of what, precisely, constituted death. The 1771 edition of the *Encyclopædia Britannica* defined death as "the separation of the soul and body; in which sense it stands opposed to life, which consists of the union thereof."[32] Likewise the *New Universal English Dictionary* defined death as "the departure of the soul from the body. Loss of sensibility, motion, and all the functions of animal life. Figuratively, the state of the dead. Murder, or depriving a person of life by violent and unlawful means. The cause of death.... In divinity, a state of insensibility, so as not to be seduced by allurements of any kind, used with unto."[33]

The advancement of the study of science and medicine during the eighteenth century built upon the theories of different scholars faster than it had in centuries past. No longer were medical philosophies dependent on the writings of the ancient scholars. Global explorations expanded the understanding of natural science and introduced new food, new plants, new animals, and new diseases into Western Europe. Research focusing on the study of death evolved in much the same way. The continued evolution of the definition of death was contingent on the research being done by academic physicians and religious scholars of the time. There were many physicians during this era who worked to identify the specific signs of death, the signs of the transition between life and death and what to do if someone had been misdiagnosed as dead. Despite the multitude of physicians working to solve this problem, the works of Drs. John Fothergill, Alexander Johnson, Charles Kite, James Curry, and Anthony Fothergill were the most prominent and were regularly quoted and cited in other sources.

The British Quaker physician, John Fothergill (1712–1780), obtained his degree in Edinburgh, where he argued in favor the common practices of blood-letting and purging. He believed that blood-letting reduced the strain on the heart because it reduced the amount of blood flowing through it. He also believed that purging assisted in the removal of mucus from the body, which would then free the nerve endings and allow the vital spirit (soul) to move more easily throughout the body.[34] He furthered his studies at London's St. Thomas Hospital, where he focused on the use of botanical pharmaceuticals. In 1744, he challenged boundaries in the medical community by becoming the first graduate from the University of Edinburgh to attain a Licentiate from the Royal College of Physicians in London.[35] Through his continued work in the medical community, he became a member of the Royal Society of Antiquities (1753), the American Philosophical Society (1776), and the Société Royale de Medicine in Paris (1776). As his personal studies advanced and his reputation gained credibility, many wealthy and titled people sought his medical services. However, when he opened his private London-based practice, the vast majority of his patients were Quakers, dissenters, and the poor. Like Culpeper before him, he did not charge a fee to those who could not afford it. Despite this, he had one of the "most lucrative private practices" in London, and his methods earned him a reputation for being a progressive and well-respected physician.[36] Fothergill challenged boundaries in the medical community, again, in 1745 when he took notice of William Tossach's essay on the resuscitative process, which had been published in Scotland the decade before. The still-growing understanding of human anatomy and physiology made the inception and use of the resuscitative process remarkable.

In 1732, the Scottish surgeon William Tossach (1700–1771) was asked to assist with the revival of miner, James Blair. Blair had been working underground and fell unconscious after being suffocated by "nauseous steam."[37] It took nearly 45 minutes for his body to be removed from the pit. When it was brought to the surface, Tossach observed that Blair's coloring was healthy, but his skin was cold and neither a pulse nor breath could be detected. By holding Blair's nose closed and blowing strongly into his mouth, Tossach was able to make Blair's chest rise. Immediately, he felt the heart begin to beat. After a pulse was detected, he opened a vein in Blair's arm and bled him for about fifteen minutes, during which time he rubbed Blair's extremities and temples, in order to help circulate the blood around the body. Finally, he applied smelling salts to Blair's nose and mouth. After about an hour, Blair began to revive and within the next four hours he was able to walk home. Unlike many medical cases from this era, Tossach included some follow up comments. He indicated that Blair was able to return to the mines within the next four days, although he "complained for a Week or two of a violent Pain in his Back."[38] Tossach believed that this pain was caused by the careless way that Blair had been removed from the mine.

J. Fothergill was so enthusiastic about the resuscitative process that he voiced his approval before London's Royal Society (for Improving Natural Knowledge) in 1744 and published his support of it in 1745. By doing so, he denoted a turning point in the study of identifying and reviving people from an apparently dead state. In his *Observations on the Recovery of a Man Dead in Appearance* (1745), Fothergill declared that this was the first time that "an artificial Inflation of the lungs ... was applied to the happy Purpose of rescuing [human] Life from such imminent Danger."[39] Stories of people being misdiagnosed as dead and reviving during their wake or after being buried had been reported since ancient times. However, the ability to test for death in a way that could also reverse the process of dying was unprecedented. The use of Tossach's method suggested that the resuscitative process could be applied to the patient in cases of suffocation, lightning strikes, drowning, and suicide by hanging. J. Fothergill surmised that this could be used in place of other commonly used resuscitation methods such as lying a person "across a Barrel Hogshead," with their head hanging down.[40] His publication of this case and its methodology made it accessible to a wide audience of medical scholars, especially throughout England. In addition, the acceptance of said process by John Fothergill likely increased its validity to other medical professionals who respected his work and opinion.

The British physician Dr. Alexander Johnson (1716–1799) believed that it was imperative to use the resuscitative process to prevent people from being buried alive. He published extensively on its successful use throughout Europe, including France, Austria, Italy, and England. Johnson's support and passion for the wide-spread use of the resuscitative process was so evident that there were times that he was mistakenly credited as being its creator. His scholarly pursuits were dedicated to identifying the signs of death and furthering the use of the resuscitative process, even going so far as to set the process to verse in 1789 so that it could be easily recalled. He identified that the resuscitative process achieved the best results when used on people who had died due to any sudden or accidental death that blocked air from entering the lungs. He impressed upon his readers that it was imperative that the resuscitative process be used immediately by whoever found the afflicted person. Waiting for a physician, medical assistant, or surgeon wasted precious time that was necessary in order to rekindle the fading "spark of life," which was believed to be the force that rekindled the soul.

Research based on the work of Descartes and Lancisi had evolved until it was theorized that the soul was responsible for keeping a person alive and for maintaining one's personality. This spark acted like a pilot light and would propel the physiological parts of the body to work on their own. A diminished spark would cause a person to slow down, and their circulatory, respiratory, and brain functions would decrease. This was believed to occur when a person appeared to be dying or was alive but lacked awareness. The person died when the spark of life blew out.

Johnson's interest in this subject came from observing that some people who were alive but appeared to be dead, a state which he described as swooning. During a swoon, a person's heart and lung functions would appear to stop working for over an hour while their body temperature gradually diminished.[41] He assured his readers that life could be recovered even when a person appeared to be so close to death by gently irritating and stimulating certain parts of the body before the resuscitative process was employed. If the person did not respond to the stimuli or the resuscitative process, then they could be "deemed absolutely dead, and may be safely consigned to the grave."[42]

In order to make certain that the resuscitative process was used as often as possible, he advocated for it to be taught to the public. Increasing awareness would allow whoever found a body to begin the process before a medical professional was called. He theorized that this would increase the number of people saved from being incorrectly diagnosed as dead and buried alive. Johnson wanted the distribution of the instructions to be overseen by the judiciary and enacted by those who were responsible for the welfare of their community: the constabulary. He feared that if the medical community controlled the administration of the practice, they would keep the knowledge for themselves.[43] This, he believed, would come at the detriment of the rest of society.

His contemporary, Charles Kite (1760–1811) was a surgeon who practiced in Kent, England. He was a member of the Company of Surgeons. His research focused on identifying the differences between apparent and absolute death. He defined apparent death as "suspended animation" or "a stoppage of the circulation, respiration, and action of the brain; the irritability, however, or that peculiar property of the muscular fibres which enables them to contract on being irritated, still remaining."[44] Absolute death was defined as "a cessation of the vital, natural, and animal functions, but where the principle of irritability is also destroyed."[45] According to Kite, the only function that separated apparent death from absolute death was "the irritability, or what has been called, the vital principle."[46] What Kite referred to as the vital principle had previously been referred to as the spark of life.

Kite included religious-based theories in his research. The words *hac animas ille evocat Orco Pallentes* adorned the title page of his *An Essay on the Recovery of the Apparently Dead* (1788). This powerful statement translated to "here souls challenge the greenish death" and referred to the soul's fight to stay inside the body and keep the person alive.[47] Stemming from the understanding that putrefaction was the only sure sign of death, the "soul's challenge" was to fight off the irreversible damage of decay. By identifying the point in time when the signs of death appeared (apparent death) and when the person could no longer be revived (absolute death), Kite enabled future research of these concepts to be either mutually inclusive or exclusive. Future scholars used Kite's definitions as the basis to discuss and refine the differences between these two stages of death. This gave them the foundation to write extensively on either concept, rather than focusing on the relatively narrow field of the connection between the two.

One such physician was Dr. James Curry (?–1819), who obtained his medical degree in Edinburgh in 1784 and became Licentiate of the Royal College of Physicians in 1801. An active supporter of the resuscitative process, he agreed with Kite's assertion that the difference between apparent death and absolute death was the status of the vital principle.[48] Adding to Kite's theories, he defined apparent death as the suspension of the body's animated functions. The person stopped breathing; their heartbeat stopped; then their body stopped moving all together, even when it was pinched, burned with fire, or pricked with needles. Despite the appearance that the body had ceased functioning, he asserted that the soul lay "dormant, and may be roused into action."[49] Once that happened, the person's health and life would be restored. Although he knew that the vital principle could remain in a dormant phase, he did not know how long it could remain that state. However, he theorized that the recovery of the vital principle was directly tied to the amount of warmth that was retained within the person's vital organs.

Just as there were circumstances where the vital principle could recover from apparent death, there were also circumstances where it could not. Cases of the latter included injuries to lungs, heart, or brain. It had not yet been identified how much force was necessary to cause irreversible damage to these organs. Therefore, Curry explained that the resuscitative process should be tried even when the person was unconscious due to injuries to any of those three organs. Rather than assuming that the person was dead, he stressed the importance of remembering "the possibility, that the person—*is not dead, but sleepeth*."[50] Once the resuscitative process had been used, the person administering the process could be assured that they had done everything in their power to ensure that the patient was absolutely dead and would not rouse after the burial process had begun.

Despite the tricky nature of the vital principle, Curry advised his readers that there were several signs that indicated that the body had transitioned into a state of absolute death. The body would grow cold and become rigid. The eyes would shrivel and sink into their sockets and the vibrancy in them would darken. The pupils of the eyes would dilate, contract, or one may dilate more than the other. If the torso or head were damaged, like when a body fell from a high place, the body could go into shock. Curry believed that such a shock could cause instant absolute death. But no matter how the person died, putrefaction was the best way to tell if a person had transitioned into the state of absolute death.

During the nineteenth century, the physician and death scholar William Tebb explained that the worst part about being misdiagnosed as dead was that the body was treated as though it was dead. This meant that once a person was proclaimed to be dead, they were not fed or given fluids. Care was not taken to ensure that the body was comfortable. They were dressed in burial clothes before their toes were sewn together, their mouths bandaged shut, and the body wrapped to be enclosed in their coffin. Their friends and families grieved for them. And, if they remained apparently dead throughout all of that, they would go through the funerary process and be buried.

James Curry's focus on the health of the vital organs is especially important as it relates to organ transplant in the modern era. Curry suggested that the resuscitative process be employed for a few hours to ensure that the person truly could not be revived before they were pronounced as dead. After that bodies were laid out and watched for up to three days in order to allow relatives and friends to say farewell and, additionally, to ensure that they were absolutely dead. Modernly, physicians and transplant teams only wait seven to ten minutes after the heart stops beating before they remove the necessary organ(s).[51] If modern practitioners waited as long as the best practices of the eighteenth century mandated, organs would not be viable for harvesting and transplantation. That said, medicine and surgery had not evolved sufficiently to allow organ transplants during the eighteenth century. Therefore, the awareness of the health of the vital organs provided a stable foundation for the more comprehensive study of the state of death, which occurred as medical theories advanced in the following centuries.

Uncertainties in identifying precisely when the body slipped into a state of absolute death caused the vast majority of premature death diagnoses. This sometimes caused people to regain consciousness even after they had been placed in what should have been their final resting place. Curry identified this and relayed the following story relating to the end of Andreas Vesalius' career.

> Vesalius the celebrated anatomist, who was physician to Charles V and to his successor Philip II, met with a similar circumstance, in the case of a Spanish nobleman whose body he was employed to open, in order to discover of what disease he had died. The nobleman's relations represented him as a murderer, and it was with difficulty that Philip rescued him from the Inquisition, upon condition that he should make a pilgrimage to Jerusalem. In returning the ship was cast away on the then desart [sic] island of Zante, where the unfortunate Vesalius perished from hunger.[52]

Although this story has since been disproven, it was a cautionary tale that was believed to be true during the eighteenth century. Additionally, there were other similar stories reported, such as the story of William Herbert, the third Earl of Pembroke who died in 1630 and whose body was removed to be embalmed. Curry reported that the Earl lifted his hand after the incision was made to open his body.[53] Unfortunately, Curry does not let the reader know what happened next, or even if the Earl survived the experience. But by retelling these stories Curry issued a warning to other doctors about what could happen if they incorrectly diagnosed someone as dead. Not only could they *cause* someone's death, but their reputations could be ruined by doing so.

Dr. Anthony Fothergill (1735–1813)—a distant relation to the aforementioned John Fothergill—was also educated in Edinburgh and graduated with his medical degree in 1763. He became a Fellow of the Royal Society in 1778 and a Licentiate of the Royal College of Physicians the following year. Over his lifetime, he also became an Honorary Member of the Medical Societies in Paris, Edinburgh, and London, and an Honorary Member of the Philosophical Societies of Manchester and Philadelphia. With such a wide array of medical and philosophical contacts, he was able to promote the effectiveness of the resuscitative process. As the eighteenth century drew to a close, he listed ways to revive people who were in the process of dying or had recently suffered a sudden or traumatic death. He believed that the resuscitative process was *an* option for revival from apparent death but not the *only* option. For example, if the person had suffocated due to "noxious air," he suggested that the air be ventilated or the person be brought outside.[54] For circumstances that violently affected the body or the mind, he suggested that "mild opiates, or Hoffman's Anodyne Liquor" be used in order to calm the body and bring it back into balance.[55] Listing the different ways that a person could be revived indicated that the resuscitative process had evolved into common practice. It was no longer the new, catch-all remedy that was used to replace the harmful techniques to dispel water from the body that had previously been used.

In addition to presenting different ways to revive a person from apparent death, A. Fothergill also suggested preventative measures to keep someone from falling into a state of apparent death to begin with. The medical community had come a long way since Queen Elizabeth I used a paste of white lead and mercury on her face to lighten her skin. By the end of the eighteenth century, the negative effects of both lead and mercury were being discussed by the medical community. A. Fothergill considered it "truly deplorable" that hard-working miners earned a pittance and were expected to "sacrifice their lives" when they worked to mine, grind, or process white lead.[56] Therefore, he suggested that masks that covered the nose and mouth be worn by laborers who regularly worked with the lead in order to prevent suffocation due to the "noxious air." He suggested that those who were exposed to the noxious vapors that came from melting lead work in well ventilated areas. If the preventative measures did not work, and a person did fall into a state of apparent death, A. Fothergill's focus turned to keeping them noticeably alive. As a practical approach, he suggested that the injured person be kept away from the location where they were injured. He also suggested that soothing music be played, or calming poetry be read in order to give their mind time to heal.

A. Fothergill warned against the early determination of death when the signs of life first disappeared. He urged his readers to continue to wait until putrefaction presented, even after the initial tests yielded no signs of life. He relayed the story of Captain Noddings, who had fallen overboard and was taken out of the water by his crew. There was no sign of life when he was examined, not even after the resuscitative process was applied. The crew was ready to toss his body overboard again but were convinced to wait until the next day. The next morning, "symptoms of *returning animation* were perceived," and he recovered soon thereafter.[57] A. Fothergill also shared the story of a sixty-year-old woman who lived in the Greenwich workhouse. She appeared to have died suddenly and was put into a coffin. The doctor was summoned and, upon viewing her, he noticed that she was still showing signs of life. Unwilling to diagnose her as dead, he returned daily, until the sixth day when she suddenly awoke and sat up in her coffin. Unfortunately, the story does not continue from there. This makes it impossible to know what caused her to fall into a state of apparent death, if she was restored to full health, or what happened afterwards.

After the bodies A. Fothergill studied progressed into a state of absolute death, he observed the stages of putrefaction. His intent was to describe each stage, so that they could be easily recognizable. He reported that the body released "carbonic acid gas," which caused the body to become clammy and take on a foul smell.[58] During the second stage of putrefaction, the body grew cold and released the putrid scent of decay. If gangrene had presented, the infection stopped spreading at this stage. A. Fothergill theorized that once these signs were evident, the living no longer had to fear prematurely burying the corpse because they understood that they were observing the finality of death.

The quest for a comprehensive definition and identification of the signs of death continued into the next century. The most notable research of the early nineteenth century was done by the Rev. Walter Whiter (1758–1832), who focused on the medical aspects of death, and British physician James Cowland Prichard (1786–1848), who focused on the evolving concept of the soul. In 1819, Whiter presented his *Dissertation on the Disorder of Death*, which built upon the work of the previously mentioned physicians. In his introduction, he stated that "I grievously fear, that the examples of revival in the Grave are more frequent than the World, amidst all their alarms existing on Premature Interment, has yet ventured to conceive."[59] Rather than presenting death as a natural part of the life process, he believed that death in and of itself was a disorder that ran against the natural process of life. He defined it as "a derangement of the System, disturbing its healthy state, in various degrees of force, from the slightest change to the condition of Death."[60] Whiter was respectful of the physicians who had worked to create a more inclusive definition of death by identifying the signs, symptoms, and stages of death during the eighteenth century. However, he apologized to his readers about the lack of progress that had been made in identifying the process of dying and making that information available to the public during the preceding century. Whiter's dissertation brought together the scholarship of many of the physicians who had sought to identify a more comprehensive definition of death and obtain a better understanding of the transition from life to death. He attempted to describe the complex and often contradictory state of the study of death at the time. As a result, his theories often contradicted those that had been developed during the eighteenth century and sometimes his own theories were fraught with internal contradictions.

By the end of the eighteenth century, certain parts of the death process could no longer be explained in simplistic terms. The signs of life were no longer considered to be a single grouping of symptoms. Instead, they were separated into two separate categories: general signs of life and signs of restored life. General signs of life included breathing, a heartbeat, pink color in the lips and cheeks, the ability to be bled from the wrists, muscles remaining soft and pliable, the ability to rouse from sleep, and the noticeable continuation of digestive, urinary, and bowel functions. In contrast, signs of restored life typically referred to twitching of the hands or mouth, mumbling, or an onlooker observing the chest of the apparently dead rising and falling as they regained the ability to breathe. As the signs and symptoms of death were being identified and cataloged, it became clear that dying was not an immediate occurrence. Rather, it was identified as a transition, where life was located at one end of the process and death at the other end.

In contrast, Whiter simplified the signs of death to "the absence of apparent motion and sensation," with the caveat that the body had also entered into a state of putrefaction.[61] Despite Kite's assertion, in 1788, that apparent death was the same state as suspended animation, the two phenomena were later identified separately. Suspended animation was considered to be the general loss of consciousness, which was sometimes accompanied by a loss of sensation or a rigidity of the body, such as when a person was in a cataleptic state. Once the person entered into a state of apparent death, tests for death would be applied to identify if the person remained in a state of apparent death or if they had transitioned to absolute death. Whiter did not agree with this theory of how a person transitioned from life to death. Instead, he theorized that the derangement of a healthy body began when apparent death presented. The difference is a matter of semantics. Previously, apparent death was considered to be the last sign of life. Here, Whiter argued that apparent death was the first sign of death. Building on the theories of Alexander Johnson, Whiter explained that there was a point in the death process where the body transitioned into an "incurable state."[62] Once the body entered into this state, any type of remedy applied to it, up to and including the resuscitative process, would no longer revive the person.

A number of other methods had been developed to restore a person back to life during the eighteenth century. The resuscitative process was enhanced and refined under the auspices of the different Humane Societies, which had been created to develop methods to restore people who presented as apparently dead due to drowning.

Several Humane Societies suggested that a person who presented as apparently dead after falling into water should be made warm by drying them and wrapping them in warm blankets with "a bladder full of warm water be placed directly on the pit of the Stomach."[63] It was considered a best practice that the recovery room should be ventilated with fresh air and that the room should be kept a comfortable temperature. The only people attending the patient should be those assisting in their treatment. An alternative to inflating the patient's lungs via mouth-to-mouth resuscitation was to use a small pair of bellows to force the pressurized air into the lungs. These bellows would be inserted into one nostril and then the other, while the mouth was held shut. When the chest rose, the medical practitioner would push the ribs back down in order to simulate breathing.

Whiter added that he believed that scrubbing the person's feet clean with a brush and briskly rubbing the soles of their feet would also be helpful if the patient was of the lower classes. He surmised that doing so would help remove calluses that had formed from years of labor and left them "less susceptible of impressions."[64] Once the callouses were removed, it would be easier for medical practitioners to stimulate the feet in an attempt to revive the person. This harkened back to a remedy from ancient times where "it was customary to apply pigeons just killed to the soles of the feet in order to rouse the Patient, [who had been] reduced to a low state of debility."[65] Whiter referred to the ancient pigeon remedy and considered it to be efficacious in extreme cases of suspended animation.

In addition to stimulating the feet, it was also important to stimulate the intestines. One of the earliest methods to do so was to blow tobacco smoke through the person's anus, in an attempt to fumigate their insides. By the nineteenth century it was more common to give an enema of salt water or water infused with peppermint oil. Once that had been completed a concoction of ammonia carbonate and olive oil was rubbed on the pulse points in an effort to stimulate them. If the patient fell into a stupor, they were sometimes bled by attaching leeches to their temples.

There was a final method of restoration, which Whiter admitted still needed further development: electricity. The theory that electricity could be used to stimulate nerves stemmed from experiments run by Luigi Galvani (1737–1798) during the 1780s. While Galvani worked at the University of Bologna, he "attached a metal rod to the legs of a dissected frog during a thunderstorm."[66] It was noticed that lightening caused the muscles within the frogs' legs to jump. Galvani theorized that this occurred because of a naturally occurring bio-electricity that he named "animal electricity." The Humane Society regularly updated the methodology of the resuscitative process; in 1798, they added the use of electricity to their process. After the body was dried, warmed, and "gently rubbed with Flannel, sprinkled with spirits or Flour of Mustard," the lungs were inflated with a small pair of bellows.[67] If the person did not rouse from sleep at this stage, it was suggested that electricity be "*early employed* by the Medical Assistants, or other judicious Practitioners" in order to stimulate the body.[68]

Reanimating the dead was of specific interest to academic physicians in England during the late eighteenth century. Due to the initial success of the Galvanic experiments Galvani's nephew, Giovanni Aldini, traveled through Europe, giving public demonstrations on the reanimation technique. After he showed this technique to a member of the Royal College of Surgeons of London (formerly the Company of Surgeons) using a decapitated dog's head, they wanted to see it done again—but using a human body. Since only the bodies of executed criminals could be legally used for this kind of medical experimentation, the body of George Foster (sometimes spelled Forrester or Forster) was used within an hour of his being hung at Newgate Prison in January 1803. The Northampton Mercury described the experiment and its value to the future of medicine:

> On the first application of the process to the face, the jaw of the deceased criminal began to quiver, and the adjoining muscles were horribly contorted, and one eye was actually opened. In the subsequent part of the process, the right hand was raised and clenched, and the legs and thighs were set in motion. It appeared to the uninformed part of the bystanders that the wretched man was on the eve of being restored to life. This, however, was impossible, as several of his friends who were under the scaffold had violently pulled his legs, in order to put a more speedy termination to his sufferings. The experiment, in fact, was of a better use and tendency. Its object was to shew [*sic*] the excitability of the human frame, when this animal electricity is duly applied. In cases of drowning or suffocation, it promises to be of the utmost use, by reviving the action of the lungs, and thereby rekindling the expiring spark of vitality. In cases of apoplexy, or disorders of the head, it offers also most encouraging prospects for the benefit of mankind.... It is the opinion of the first medical men, that this discovery, it rightly managed and duly prosecuted, cannot fail of great, and perhaps, as yet, unforeseen utility.[69]

While giving each of the other methods of restoration the credit that he believed they deserved, Whiter encouraged the use of the resuscitative process in addition to those suggestions, even after the body had begun to show signs of death. He believed that Galvanism had potential to be used to restore life to a dead person in the future but admitted that science had not evolved to that point yet. Therefore, he strongly urged that means of restoration and resuscitation in the case of "all cases of Death, under all circumstances, and upon all occasions."[70]

Whiter also hypothesized about factors that could be strong enough to cause the cessation of the vital principle. It was already understood that vital principle did not follow the laws of physics or chemistry. The accepted theory during the early nineteenth century was that if the person remained in a state of apparent death without decaying, the vital principle was still active. Whiter believed that people died from fevers because poison lurked within their bodies. He further theorized that this poison could have been the initial cause of the fever or it could have been "a Putrid matter generated in the course of the Fever."[71] This poison was believed to be so powerful that it caused the fluids within the body to decay, which would then affect the nervous system and cause the vital principle to wither away.

As previously identified, theories of religion and medicine were interrelated. Therefore, academic physicians of the time needed to incorporate religious beliefs into the definition of death for it to be considered medically viable. Leading into the middle of the nineteenth century, Dr. James Prichard continued the work of Kite and Whiter when he wrote his *Review of the Doctrine of a Vital Principle* (1829). Prichard had achieved his medical degree at the University of Edinburgh in 1808 before settling in Bristol, England. He became a Fellow of the Royal Society in 1827. Prichard explained that historically the vital principle had been viewed as "a real entity, a sort of in-dwelling guardian of the body."[72] This guardian was responsible for maintaining the functions of the body that kept it in good health. When the soul was disturbed, it created disorder within the body. Then it would follow its instinct to restore the body's "healthful and regular conditions."[73] However, despite the many experiments and operations that had been done on countless bodies, there had not been any evidence of the soul residing within it. In response, Prichard theorized that the vital principle was not a metaphysical essence of life, alertness, and/or the personality. Instead, he believed that the vital principle was a physiological substance; specifically, the electric fluid, which he theorized ran between the nerves of the body, carrying their impulses from one nerve to the next.

Proof of this theory had been evident in William Buchan's *Domestic Medicine* (1774). William Buchan (1729–1805) was a physician who concerned himself with bringing simple, yet effective, medicine to the general public. Initially published in Scotland (1769), over 145 editions of his *Domestic Medicine* books were published and reissued until the final printing in Philadelphia (1871). His books were published in English, rather than Latin, in an easily identifiable chapter format. In his chapter "On Casualties," he explained that no one should be "looked upon as killed by any accident, unless where the structure of the heart, brain, lungs, or some organ necessary to life is evidently destroyed."[74] And even then, the person responsible for determining death in the injured person needed to wait until the body grew cold in order to ensure that the person would not revive. Buchan's books exemplified the importance of the bringing academic level research to the common person. He believed that such important information should not have been known by only the elite few. By publishing information like the signs of death and what to do when someone appeared to have died, he helped disseminate this information to the general public.

There has been a considerable amount of modern research done on the expansion of the definition of death, with a particular focus on post–1960s brain death, organ death, and cell death. When the ad hoc committee at Harvard Medical School came together to decide if an irreversible coma would count as a new criterion for death, they identified that the "current" criteria included "a total stoppage of the circulation of the blood, and cessation of the animal and vital functions consequent there upon such as respiration, pulsation, etc."[75] These indicators were signs of death that had been observed and recorded by doctors throughout the eighteenth century. Updated criterion to define death in the United States consists of "an individual who has sustained either (1) irreversible cessation of circulator and respirator functions or (2) irreversible cessation of all functions of the entire brain, including the brainstem."[76] However, the criterion for death in the United Kingdom requires test results that show the "irreversible cessation of functioning of the brain stem."[77] The doctors of the eighteenth century also put particular emphasis on the importance of the brain and knew that an injury to it could cause a person to fall unconscious, into a coma, or appear to have died altogether. This, too, shows echoes in the modern understanding of brain death, which is described as "a person who has irreversibly lost all clinical functions of the brain."[78]

CHAPTER 4

The Burial Process
and Premature Repercussions

"A Woman was buried at St. Catharine's Church and a Noise being heard in the Night and next Morning in the Grave, the Coffin was taken up and open'd, when the Woman was found to be alive, but very bloody and much bruised; yet she lived but a few hours after, and was again buried the next Night."[1]

* * *

By the eighteenth century, it was understood that death was "an irreversible condition."[2] The process of how death overtook life remained a mystery, however. Although medical scholars theorized about the transition from life to death, their theories were not well-known by people outside of the scholarly medical and religious communities. This meant that most people did not know how to identify the different stages of oncoming death, or when a body was apparently dead vs. absolutely dead, or when revival might still be possible. The concept of someone being simultaneously alive and dead was not generally accepted. Theories to define death were developed to provide clarity about the transitional stages between life and death. Additionally, physicians within the medical community worked with the administration of their respective cities and published books on the resuscitative process. Philosophy intertwined with religious and medical theories causing debates on whether death was an interruption of life, or if life was an interruption of death.

People continued to be misdiagnosed as dead during the Enlightenment, just as they had been during the Middle Ages and Renaissance. Stories of people waking up after being incorrectly diagnosed as dead were published in books, pamphlets, and newspapers, which had readership bases ranging from academic scholars to the general public of the United Kingdom. After being misdiagnosed as dead, the person was either prematurely enclosed in their coffin, buried, interred, or dissected before

70

they woke up again. In order to condense these consequences into an easily identifiable phrase, I developed the term "premature repercussion(s)." As people continued to suffer premature repercussions as a consequence of being incorrectly diagnosed as dead, the medical community realized that the accepted tests for death were not as effective as they had hoped. As the signs of life and death continued to be identified, tests to confirm them were enhanced, refined, and adapted to correspond with updated anatomical, physiological, and spiritual theories. It became imperative that whoever diagnosed a person as absolutely dead ensured that the person had both exited from their current state and entered into the next stage of their transition from life to death.

In 1789, the *Kentish Gazette* published an article that discussed options that were under debate by the medical community regarding how precisely to do this. It was assumed that the body progressed from unconscious stage of suspended animation to apparent death when the body lost the ability to propel the blood through the circulatory system and then grew cold.[3] When this occurred, medical professionals would have the option of either allowing the body to achieve apparent death, or attempting to draw the body back into a state of suspended animation. In order to cause the body to reverse the course of death, the most important objective was to restore the person's body temperature. Some antiquarian physicians believed that the best way to adjust the natural heat within the body was to submerse it into cold water. However, practitioners during the eighteenth century preferred to prescribe stimulants, such as the "vapour of the spirit of sal armoniac [*sic*]," otherwise known as ammonium chloride, which was used for smelling salts.[4] Critics of this theory pointed out that these stimulants only helped a person regain consciousness; they did not restimulate the body's core temperature. Additionally, there were concerns about the safety of inhaling sal ammoniac into the lungs due to its poisonous nature. However, since such smelling salts were commonly used to rouse women who had fainted—and fainting was considered to be a type of suspended animation—it was believed that the vapor of sal ammoniac was a credible substance to revive people who had fallen into a state of suspended animation in general.

There were several common diagnostic techniques that a medical professional or an aware citizen would have at their disposal if a person seemed to have transitioned from a state of apparent death into absolute death. Basic tests for death attempted to elicit a response based on sensory or automatic body functions. Respiration was tested by putting a mirror or a piece of glass up to the person's nose or mouth to see if it fogged. If such an item could not be procured, a candle would be lit and held similarly. The flame would be watched to see if the person's breath caused it to move.[5]

As time progressed, it became preferable to hold fine wool or cotton up to the person's face rather than using fire. Not only were the tests done with candles dangerous, but they sometimes caused incorrect results. Additionally, using fire to rouse someone during a time when mattresses were made out of straw and homes were made out of wood, stone, or brick without any fire retardant in the walls, floor, or ceiling, could have catastrophic results. The type of object used did not matter, however, since this test was reported as yielding false positive results and the body started to decay over time rather than reviving.[6] The olfactory sense would be tested by holding pungent scented items under the person's nose.[7] It was expected that the strong smell would cause the body to respond in the same way as it would if sal ammoniac been used. Early circulatory tests included blistering or burning the skin in order to stimulate the blood and see if the person would react to the intense pain. If the person responded to any of the tests, they were considered to be alive and were treated as though they would recover.[8] Recovery treatment included bed rest, keeping the patient warm, and stimulating their arms and legs to aid blood flow and muscle movement. However, if the patient did not respond to the stimulation tests, they were assumed to have transitioned into a state of absolute death, at which time the burial process would begin.

Causing pain was used as a general way to test if a person was in an apparently dead state. Boiling water, melted wax, or the flame of a lit match would be used to try to startle people and transition them back to life. Their fingers or toes would be stabbed with pins in order to see if the muscles would twitch or the person would regain consciousness with a gasp or shout. In some cases, hot irons were place on the top of a person's head in an attempt to elicit a response. In his treatise *De Subitaneis Mortibus* (1707), Lancisi explained that "some labouring People, who could not by the most strong and powerful Remedies be oused [sic] from profound Apoplexies have been instantly restored to Life by applying hot Irons to the Soles of their Feet."[9] His support of such extreme remedies could have been a consequence of being misdiagnosed as dead during his childhood. Having been through the revival process, himself, after falling into an apparently dead state, he may have retained legitimate concerns about accidentally diagnosing someone as dead and burying them alive.

It is easy to wonder if any of these tests were actually used, especially those that seem inhumane. The same tests were referenced as being used across Western Europe indicating that they were used extensively, plausibly because they yielded accurate results. More definitively, in 1997, Georges Leonetti and his team from the Université de la Méditerranée published their findings regarding the use of pin implementation to test for death during the 1722 plague outbreak in France. Approaching the study from an anthropological perspective, the team studied 200 human skeletons that were removed from a mass grave in Marseilles. Two of the skeletons had bronze pins embedded into the bone at the top of the big toe. Based on the placement of the pins, the team hypothesized that "the pin had been introduced under the big toenail."[10] The presence of these pins helps give validity to the idea that the rest of the tests for death were also practiced. Had only one or two tests for death worked, it would have been much easier—and in the case of printing costs, cheaper—to reprint only the revival techniques that had favorable results. Likewise, if none of the tests ever worked, it would have been medically acceptable and religiously viable to give credence to God's will.

However, even the clergy were not willing to blame God for every death. Instead, they worked in conjunction with the medical community to educate the public about what happened to the body and soul after death. Just as Charles Kite had included religious theory in his medical-based definition of death, the eighteenth-century minister John Bowden referred to medical theory in his *Sermon ... at the Funeral of Mr. James Blunt* (1749). He explained that the body was considered to be a vessel that carried the soul. Therefore, he considered the "life of the body" and the life of the soul to be two separate constructs.[11] Blending the religious debate of the soul with medical theory of the time, he postulated that the body's perception of the world shifted as the body decayed and that this would cause only the spirit to remain. Bowden included two signs of life (breathing and the soul) into the following question from Genesis 2:7, which he posed to his listeners: "Is it not he that first breathed into Man's Nostrils the vital Flame, and who constantly maintains it?"[12] Unlike many philosophers of the time who believed that death was something that happened to a person, Bowden personified death and gave it a purpose. Explaining how death affected the body, he postulated that "Death breaks the Springs of Life; extinguishes the Spirits; stagnates the Blood; puts an End to all vital and animal Action; crumbles us to dust and dissolves the close knit Union between Body and Soul."[13] Likewise, he gave an awareness to the corpse, describing the surprise that it must have felt as it transitioned from a living, breathing person who was able to talk with others, to losing all capability, as the coloration of the skin paled and life ebbed away. But when the life of the body ceased, the life of the soul began and entered "into the World of Spirits, [where] a new and amazing Scene of Things open'd to its view."[14] He theorized that when death came, it freed the soul and allowed it to have a better life than it did while it was contained within the body. To this end, he considered the grave to be a house for a corpse. He found it fitting that the human corpse resided in houses made of the earth, particularly because humans had come from the earth. Like the doctors who described death in transitional phases, Bowden described death as a passageway for a new and "unknown state."[15]

Due to the work being done by the medical community, the stories being published in the British press, and their own experiences, the public was aware that people were being incorrectly diagnosed as dead and suffering premature repercussions. The medical community did not deny that these issues were occurring and continued to develop theories to accurately diagnose people as dead. The British press published a variety of articles about the circumstances regarding those who woke during the watching period or were found mangled inside of the coffin or huddled into the corner of their tombs. They reported on the use of the resuscitative process to awaken people who appeared to have died due to suffocation, strangulation, or drowning. With each story, the British public were able to read about the horrible repercussions that befell those who had the misfortune to be improperly diagnosed as dead. One such story was that of 80-year-old Mrs. Fudge from Cornwall, England. As she lay dying, she insisted that there be a two-day delay between the time she was declared dead and when she was buried. After she passed, her body began to be prepared for burial. As the preparations continued, someone noticed that the middle of her back felt warm. In response, her friends put a mirror up to her mouth. But after repeated attempts did not show any respiration on the mirror, her body was laid out in a room with the windows open. That evening her body temperature began to rise and, finally, those assembled noticed that she was breathing.[16]

An Abridged History of Burial in the United Kingdom

The way that the corpse was treated and the accouterments that it was buried with evolved over time. When the authority of Rome collapsed in Britain during the fifth century, burial customs began to shift. Depending on the social-status of the dead, the Anglo-Saxon pagans (of the fifth and sixth centuries) buried their dead with goods that they might need in the afterlife. Those with the highest social-statuses could be buried with clothing and accessories, tools, weaponry and even food. Warriors may have been buried with their clothes, weaponry, and—although rarely—their horse. In 1997, a team of archaeologists were excavating at the Royal Air Force base in Lakenheath, Suffolk (RAF Lakenheath), in search of the remains of early Anglo-Saxons. Over the course of the dig (1997–2001), they excavated three cemeteries, which included 435 burials and more than 17 cremated remains.[17] One of the people buried was a warrior, whose grave included a shield, a sword, and a spear, as well as his horse, a bridal, a bucket, and "cuts of sheep."[18] Common people were buried with what they had; in some cases men were buried with their weaponry and women were buried with jewelry or tools to make fiber arts. In other cases, people were not buried with any goods at all.

Christian burial culture evolved alongside those of the Anglo-Saxons. During the sixth century, Christian missionaries began to associate with Anglo-Saxons with the goal of converting them to Christianity. The graves of saints were identified, and churches were built around those graves and named for them. The ground that they were buried on was considered to be holy, and people continued to be buried in those cemeteries. As parishes developed and conversions to Christianity increased, it became the duty of the priests to commit the dead to their graves. As the Middle Ages progressed, Christian burials became the predominant customs.

By the fourteenth century, the wake had become normalized as part of the burial process in England. As the life of a dying person waned, a priest came to administer last rites. These happened in three parts. First, the priest would hear the dying person's confession and absolution would be granted. After this, the priest would request God's forgiveness by performing their last anointing of the sick, otherwise called the sacrament of extreme unction. Finally, a consecrated wafer would be put into the person's mouth as a provision for their journey into death. Once a person was committed to their deathbed, friends and family came to watch for signs that the process of death had completed. After the family was certain that death was absolute, the corpse would be washed and wrapped in a shroud with the top and the bottom knotted or the sides sewn shut. If the family were impoverished, the preparation process would end there and the person would be buried only in their shroud. Those in the merchant class may have been able to afford a hand-made coffin and the shrouded corpse would have been placed inside prior to burial. In these cases, there was often a parade of friends, family, guild members, and other associates who brought the body from the bier to the cemetery. The wealthy had more choices when it came to the burial of their dead, including embalming the corpse or moving the body to another location altogether.

Relocating a body for burial before the age of refrigeration meant that there were limited means of halting the decomposition of the body. If the death had occurred recently, and the body needed to be transported somewhere less than three days away, it could be embalmed. In the Middle Ages, embalming a body consisted of opening the torso and cleaning out the innards with vinegar to keep the organs from rotting. Once cleaned, the body cavity would be filled with salt and different spices to mask some of the smell of decay. After the torso was sewn back together, strips of wax-dipped linen would be wrapped around the body. If the body was wrapped well enough, it could be dressed before it was transported to the place where it would be buried. If the body needed to travel a longer distance, there was no way to stop it from decaying in transit. Therefore, the insides would be removed, and the body would be dismembered and boiled in order to separate the flesh and muscles from the skeleton. The flesh and muscles would then be buried in the location where the person had died, and the bones would be taken to the preferred place of burial.

It was believed that once the body and the soul had separated, the usefulness of the body had come to an end. The lifeless shell of the body was considered "abhorrent," and it was considered poor form to keep the body anywhere that it could poison people in its general vicinity.[19] A body could not be kept inside the house beyond the time of the wake, otherwise it might infect the rest of the family. Nor could it be put outside or thrown into a local fresh water supply, otherwise the poison from the decay could taint the surrounding area. In order to save the living from the dead, there was clear message of "stay down there," as the body was put into a grave and covered with tightly packed dirt so that neither the smell nor the body itself could rise again.[20]

The sixteenth century was a tumultuous one for England. During plague years, there was a two- to three-day lapse between the time the person died and when they were buried. The plague orders of 1583 had indicated that the bodies of those who died of plague could not be kept inside of a church while public assemblies or services were in session.[21] The responsibility to bury the dead primarily fell to the individual parishes, who managed the burials by acquiring new locations for the burials to take place, situating the graves, and collecting associated fees.[22] The city administration only stepped in when the parish could no longer manage the number of bodies they were responsible for burying. When the plague broke out in London, the city's approximately 125 parishes could not manage the burial of the tens of thousands of people who died. The number of burials necessary severely stressed each parish's resources, both in manpower to remove and bury the bodies and in finding physical locations for those bodies to be buried. Specifically during the plague years, when parish cemeteries and overflow burial grounds ran out of space, or time, bodies were buried together in mass graves, which were covered with dirt when they became full.

To allow for people to be buried in a parish churchyard, overflow burial grounds were engineered. These burial grounds were initially created on one acre of city land in the Moorlands part of London, on which Bethlem Hospital was located. In 1569, the New Churchyard burial ground was established as a precautionary measure. The city administration was

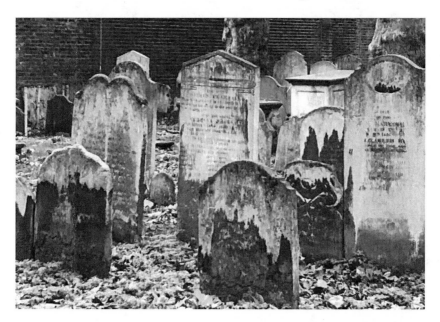

Old graves from Bunhill Burial Grounds in London, England (photograph by the author).

concerned that if there was another outbreak of disease, there would not be enough room to bury the dead in the existing space. In the end, the idea to create this site turned out to be good one. It was used for many years and the ground was saturated with bodies during the plague of 1665. The success of the creation of New Churchyard burial ground was used as precedence for new burial grounds to be created after the original ones were no longer usable. In response, the city of London chose to build a new burial ground on Bunhill Fields during the plague of 1665. Bunhill Fields Burial Grounds was not consecrated and was used to bury dissenters and radicals after the plague had subsided.

Burial culture during the seventeenth century was dependent on the person's religion. Traditionalist Christians, for example, believed that the body should be handled honorably and the burial celebrations should be grand. Similarly, Richard Hooker, an Anglican priest, surmised that the purpose of the funeral was for the living to show their love for the recently deceased and their hope that they would be resurrected when the time came.[23] Puritans and some Protestants were of the mind that it was more important to have a simple burial. After being tended to at home, the body would be taken to burial location and be "immediately interred without any ceremony."[24]

Since the accepted religious practices of the time changed with the monarchs, it became both imperative and difficult for people to stay in the good graces of the church. Running afoul of the church could mean more than the end of a person's life. It could also follow them into the afterlife. Since the responsibility of burial fell to the churches, they also had the right not to give people a proper and honorable burial. In these cases, the bodies were buried within the boundaries of the parish but not on consecrated ground. One did not necessarily have to be a murderer of another or of oneself (suicide) to be ostracized from an honorable burial. Babies who died before baptism were treated with the utmost indignity because they were considered to be "less than human."[25] This often resulted in their bodies being buried in a "secret place" where the body would be kept safe from animals.[26]

* * *

Culture regarding the burial process was in flux during the eighteenth century. After a person was declared to be dead, the body was cleaned and made presentable for the friends and family to visit the body. In order to properly prepare the person for viewing, it was mandatory that the deceased's eyes be dealt with first. This was due to a popular omen that a corpse whose eyes would not close represented "a threat to its kin."[27] Since this would have been noticed while the corpse was being viewed, those who prepared the body used pennies to weight the corpses' eyes closed. Historic concerns about the corpse being a threat to their family may could have been because the person who returned from the grave was hostile about their nearly permanent burial or interment.

After the eyes had been properly closed, the mouth was shut, and the jaw was held in place by a wide band which wrapped around the chin. Next, the arms were folded across the corpse's stomach or chest, and the legs were straightened. In order to keep the legs straight, the ankles were tied together with bands of fabric. These bands would be cut prior to burial, so that the spirit could easily be resurrected at the time of the Reckoning.[28] Once the corpse was ready, it would be dressed either in a shroud or a winding sheet and placed in the coffin to be displayed. Those who could afford it had access to a "growing range of funerary products: shrouds, coffins, hearses, escutcheons (coats of arms), rings, mourning clothes, and so on."[29] In all cases, it was imperative to watch the corpse because not adhering to burial rituals could cause lasting repercussions for the dead—especially the apparently dead.

Once the corpse was properly prepared and dressed, it was customary to watch the body until the time of the funeral. Historic and growing concerns of a premature diagnosis of death caused customs such as watching the corpse during the wake to become commonplace. The tradition of waking, or "the wake" began in the fourteenth century. At that time, the purpose was to watch for the signs that death was imminent, so that a priest could be summoned at the appropriate time. By the eighteenth century, the priest was summoned after the person appeared to have died. From that point until the funeral, the body was watched for signs of life. Movement, a gasp for air or a steady breath, even the flickering of eyelids or twitching of fingers or toes could signify that the person being watched was reviving. Watching the body allowed for the emergence of decay, which was understood to be the only certain sign that the person was absolutely dead. It also fulfilled the belief that the noise and the light made by the visitors would protect "the body from evil spirits."[30]

The grandeur and location of the wake was dependent on the social status of the family of the deceased. It was customary for guests to receive "a few glasses of mulled wine both before leaving the deceased's house and on return from the church."[31] Funerals of the poor were paid for by their local parish, and the gatherings were generally modest. Their homes were small, so the body was placed in the center of the main room. Wealthy families could afford to have larger parties complete with food and drink. The corpse would be placed in the middle of the room so that the guests could look upon the deceased as they feasted.[32] The location of the wake shifted throughout the eighteenth century. Initially, the body was kept in a larger room, but by the middle of the century it was kept out of the way in a little used room with one person watching over it. In the latter case, the body would often be left alone, which entirely defeated the purpose of the wake.

The length of time that the body was supposed to be watched prior to burial has traditionally been reported as three days, although there were no laws specifically mandating the length of time in England. The necessity of waiting until the body had started to decompose had worked its way into English burial customs, and it was considered indecent and disrespectful of the dead to forgo laying the corpse out to be watched.[33] Using modern science, we can theorize that the idea of a three-day waiting period came about because "the beginning stages of putrefaction can be observed after 48–72 hours."[34] In the simplest terms, putrefaction is "the bacterially induced breakdown of soft tissue and subsequent alteration of their protein, carbohydrate and fat constituents."[35]

The importance of watching the body during the wake was indicated in the March 12, 1791, edition of the *Ipswich Journal*:

> David Bach, a painter, travelling through Germany, was suddenly taken ill, and apparent death took place. His servants who watched his corpse after it was lain out, endeavoured [sic] to console themselves with the bottle. As they grew elevated, one of them proposed giving his old master a glass of liquor,

which he had been far from having a dislike to when alive: this was accordingly done, and the consequence was, that he recovered and lived many years.[36]

Likewise, in 1787, Isaac Rooke had recently been discharged by St. Bartholomew's Hospital (London). Soon after, he decided to visit his brother in Chesterfield, Derbyshire, located approximately 150 miles north of London. He was found in an apparently dead state, in an unnamed town along his route. His body was laid out in St. Peter's Church, at which time the coroner and a jury were sent for to watch over the body. Just as they were leaving, one of the people noticed his stomach move. They felt for his pulse and noticed that it beat strongly. He was removed and set up in a public house, where he was put into a warm bed and "proper methods [were] used for his recovery."[37] By the following Friday, he had recovered well enough to continue his journey.

This was not the first time that Rooke had this experience. After his recovery, he explained that he was given to convulsive fits and that doctors had tried to remedy the problem by bleeding him to calm him down. Only a few weeks prior, Rooke had been so affected by a fit that he lay apparently dead in his coffin, while his funeral arrangements were made. At that time, someone had seen him breathing, and he was saved from the "unhappy" circumstance of being buried alive.[38] After his most recent episode, he began carrying a letter in his pocket which explained both his medical condition and how it should be treated.

Despite the delay in burial and the care taken to watch the body, people continued to be misdiagnosed as dead and suffer the consequences of premature repercussions. According to Jean-Benigne Winslow, an eighteenth-century physician with a particular interest in the prematurely buried, the ancient physicians who dealt with the problem of premature burial advised that educated individuals use all "possible Methods of recalling the Dead to Life" and continue to look for new methods to do so.[39] By reprinting this ancient request in his book at the beginning of the eighteenth century, he reminded the medical community of the plea from the ancient scholars. Fortuitously, Winslow's book was published during the same decade as John Fothergill's book in support of the resuscitative process. The close proximity of the publication dates between the two books may have contributed to the medical community's interest in using the resuscitative process to decrease the amount of people being prematurely buried.

When it came to the actual burial of the body, the economic differences became more apparent. Most bodies were buried in parish churchyards, yet depending on the socio-economic class, they were buried differently. The poor were more likely to wrap their dead in linen or muslin cloth. The parish may have had a coffin that they could loan the family to bring the body from the wake to the burial. Once there, the body would be deposited directly into the ground, without the protection of the coffin. The poorest of people were buried in "poors' holes." These were open pits in certain parish cemeteries which remained open until they were full, at which time they were covered with dirt. By the end of the eighteenth century, a more formal funeral for a poor person could cost as much as £15, the equivalent of over three months' salary for a skilled tradesman.[40]

Families with more financial resources could afford to have their loved ones buried in coffins. In some cases, families chose the cost-effective assurance of keeping the family together by burying them in the same coffin. Those of the subjectively middle class or lower gentry could bury their dead in smaller churchyards located in the suburban areas of the bigger cities. Rather than burying their dead in the ground, the rich had the ability to finance the burial of their dead in vaults, shafts, mausoleums, or inside church catacombs. In these cases, the structures were often lined with bricks or stone in order to protect the body from being moved or crowded and allowed the family to control access to the bodies that were buried there. Other options included burying their families in small, private, graveyards, vaults, or "brick-lined shafts" that were not attached to a church.[41] The rich also had the ability to hire people to guard the place where they had chosen to bury their family. The guards would be responsible for ensuring that the recently buried would stay that way, remaining safe from resurrectionists. These guards were also responsible for listening for sounds from the grave, ensuring that those who had been buried were actually dead.

Once the body was buried, it was no longer the family's concern. In accordance with the burial laws of the eighteenth century, a buried corpse was considered to be abandoned property. This left the body vulnerable to disinterment by the resurrectionists. Despite the stealthy techniques that were used to disinter bodies, their work was one of the worst kept secrets in England. Both the public and the medical community were well aware of what was happening. Those involved with the medical community were acutely aware of the situation because they were intrinsically linked to it. The growth of medical schools and an interest in studying medicine, anatomy, and surgery, caused the demand for cadavers to rise. In the Lambeth section of London, a gang of resurrectionists charged "six shillings for the first foot, and nine [pence] per inch" for children's bodies and "two guineas and a crown" for adult bodies.[42] The approximate equivalency of the cost of an adult body in 2020 was approximately £287 and a starting rate of around £37 for a child's body.[43] Preference was given to fresh bodies, as well as bodies with anatomical differences. These differences could have been as normal as pregnancy or as different as malformations. As the demand for cadavers continued, resurrectionists raised the prices of the bodies that they supplied.[44] Administrators for medical schools and hospitals, the practitioners, and students had no choice but to pay the prices that were demanded. Additionally, if school administrators did not pay the resurrectionists, they risked losing students to professors who could adequately supply their students with the bodies necessary for their anatomical studies.

Aside from the fact that only a few bodies could be retrieved legally, buying bodies from resurrectionists was more cost efficient than picking up a body from an execution, even though the body itself was free. The Royal College of Physicians is in possession of two receipts from 1694 which included the costs for transporting a body from the gallows to the College. These receipts include a detailed account of the costs for transportation of the body, assistance, washing the operating theater, drinks, and supplies, as well as line items for the coffin, cleaning the fabric that the body was wrapped in, and the burial of the body. The final associated costs were £2.15.8 (pounds/shillings/pence) and £3.14.3, respectively. This had the approximate 2020 equivalency of £597 and £797.[45]

When the deceased were not guarded or protected in private graveyards, it left them vulnerable to resurrectionists. Once the body became the property of the resurrectionists, one could never be certain where that body would be taken or who it would be used by. Sometimes bodies were taken from outside of London and brought to the different medical schools or practitioners. Other times bodies were removed from the cemeteries or graveyards in London. One such case was presented by James Blake Bailey, who published the remains of a resurrectionist's diary at the end of the nineteenth century.

> There is a case on record of a child who had died of scrofula, and whose body was brought to St. Thomas' Hospital by Holliss, a well-known resurrectionist. The body was at once recognized by one of the students as that of his sister's child; on this being made known to the authorities at the hospital, the corpse was immediately buried before any dissection had taken place.[46]

Resurrectionists and the Medical Narrative

Let it never be said that people are not resourceful. If there is a shortage of a commodity, there will be someone who will decide to make that commodity their trade. The need to procure bodies for medical professionals gave rise to resurrectionism. Specifically, this was the action of taking a corpse from the grave to be sold to the medical community for the purpose of dissection. This practice became an instrumental part of the medical community. Without the bodies supplied by the resurrectionists, medical practitioners would not have been able to perform intricate anatomical studies. Nor would they have been able to conduct multiple tests of their theories on bodies before they were used on living people. These tests were imperative to advance the theories and boundaries of scientific medicine during the eighteenth and nineteenth centuries.

Modern scholarship regarding the study of death during the eighteenth and early nineteenth centuries has typically focused on the evolution of burial customs, the evolution of medical theory, and the sale of the corpse. Initial analyses have shown a call and response pattern between society and the medical community, where society noticed a problem and then turned to the medical community to provide a solution. Part of the medical narrative was also shaped by the resurrectionists who exhumed and sold recently buried bodies to medical schools for profit. Resurrectionists entered the medical narrative after the tests for death had verified that a person was absolutely dead and the body had been buried or interred. Very soon after the burial, usually the same night, the resurrectionists would dig up the grave and remove the body. Once they had possession of the body, it would then be sold to a medical school, physician, surgeon, anatomist, or medical student.

The *New Universal Etymology and Pronouncing Dictionary* (1848) defined a resurrectionist as "one who exhumes dead bodies by stealth, for the purpose of dissection."[47] This definition aligned with a story from the *Sussex Advertiser*, which was published nearly a century earlier:

> On Thursday last the Churchwardens of the Parish of St. Giles's in the Fields indicted one Thomas Hayes at Hicks's Hall, for taking dead Bodies out of the several Church-Yards in and about Town, and selling them to Surgeons. The Court sentenced him to be confined six Months in Newgate, and to pay a certain Fine. The Court declared their great Dislike to such unnatural Behaviour, and will punish it more severely for the future.[48]

Some historians have favored the term "body-snatcher" over the use of the word "resurrectionist," and sometimes the words have been used interchangeably in both historical and modern scholarship. However, there are distinctions between the two terms. The most prominent difference was how they were used during the eighteenth century. While the term "resurrectionist" was typically used to depict a job title, the term "body-snatching" was often used to explain what resurrectionists did— they snatched bodies from their graves. When the term body-snatching was changed to denote the job title, it changed the tone of the trade. Rather than being a valid, necessary part of the medical community, those who were employed to carry out these duties seemed underhanded and nefarious. They became 'the other': the person who was not like the general law abiding British citizen. A mock advertisement published in the October 29, 1811, edition of the *Morning Post*, played on this concept. The tongue-in-cheek article described issues that were decided upon at the "general meeting of the Gentlemen in the *resurrection* line, vulgarly called '*body snatchers*,' '*dead carcase* [sic] *stealers*,' &c."[49] The concept of body-snatching was also mentioned in news reports, such as this article from the December 9, 1817, issue of the *Hull Packet*:

> The depositories of the dead have been nightly invaded, and the feelings of surviving relatives exceedingly harrowed, by the depredations upon their deceased friends, of that callous gang of wretches known by the name of Body Snatchers whose industry in their disgusting trade has been particularly exercised in the new burial-ground at Lambeth.... [The sexton] accordingly hired two men, and instructed them to be vigilant; still the ground was robbed; scarcely a night passed without a body being stolen, and yet the offenders were not discovered.[50]

Around that same time, the term body-snatcher began to become ambiguous. An article from the *Morning Advertiser* (1818) reported an argument that had arisen when four men took a cart that belonged to a "Sherriff's officer," then asked that he pay to get it back. As they began to bicker back and forth the officer called them "night-robbers," and, in return, they declared that he "was a body snatcher, who had come with his cart to carry away dead and live bodies...."[51] A few years earlier, students of St. Thomas's Hospital brought charges against six "well-known resurrection-men" who had increased the price of bodies from four guineas to six guineas.[52] The article specifically equated the two terms by stating that they were "known by the vulgar appellation of resurrection-men or *body snatchers*."[53] Despite the ambiguity of the term body-snatcher, the social definition of the term resurrectionist remained stable throughout the eighteenth and nineteenth centuries, and thus is the primary term used in this book.

Bransby Blake Cooper's biography of his uncle, Sir Astley Cooper, provided a generally normalized view on the profession of resurrectionism during the eighteenth century. Sir Astley was a British anatomist and surgeon, whose research furthered the study of a variety of areas of anatomy and physiology, including vascular surgery, hand surgery, and orthopedic surgery, as well as the pathology of the human ear, testicles, mammary glands, and abdominal wall hernias. Sir Astley Cooper started his day by meeting with the resurrectionists who were interested in working for him. He reviewed the bodies that they had disinterred during the evening and chose those that he believed would serve him best. In some cases, he used the acquired cadavers while he taught anatomy at St. Thomas's Hospital. Other times, he used them for his personal studies. B.B. Cooper described his uncle's relationship with the resurrectionists as the following:

> [he] had to mix himself with a set of persons who were at that time essential to him, as to all other teachers of Anatomy and Surgery, to enable them to perform the duties which they had undertaken. I allude to the men whose occupation was to procure Subjects for dissection, since known by the name of Resurrectionists.[54]

The relationship between the medical community and the resurrectionists resulted in the evolution of the understanding of the signs, stages, and definition of death. Concurrently, the medical community had a shortage of cadavers for their anatomical dissections, so they relied on the resurrectionists to obtain the freshest cadavers available. This culminated in two sets of resurrectionist gangs (one in England, one in Scotland) who turned to murder to fulfill the requests during the 1820s and 1830s. This shocking turn of events broke the trust between the medical community and public society. Medical practitioners and administrators no longer trusted the resurrectionists. The public feared anatomists and that the resurrectionists who worked for them would murder them for their corpses. The tenuous relationship resulted in legal changes regarding how the medical community legally obtained their cadavers. This ultimately brought the era of publicly acceptable resurrectionism to a close in 1832.

CHAPTER 5

The Corpse as a Commodity in a Changing World

It has been said that the French novelist Abbé Prevost had an apoplectic fit and to all appearances died in Chantilly Forest during the fall of 1763. He was taken to a nearby village, and an autopsy was performed. When he screamed as his body was being opened, the surgeon realized that Prevost was not absolutely dead. Unfortunately, the wounds sustained by the autopsy were too severe to survive and he died from his injuries.[1]

* * *

The dissolution of the Company of Barber Surgeons, in 1745, led to the foundation of the Company of Surgeons. This new professional association provided grants for dental students, funding for poverty-stricken surgeons and barbers, and supported "the teaching of anatomy at the Royal College of Surgeons."[2] It also allowed surgeons to perform dissections without the Company's approval. Around this time, people became more interested in receiving a formalized medical education, especially in London. Continuing to build on the foundation of hands-on learning that had been set in place by Paracelsus, Vesalius, and Harvey, the use of cadavers helped advance the study of anatomy by empirical observation rather than theoretical study. As the interest in medical education increased, so too did the need for cadavers. John Abernethy, a surgeon working at St. Bartholomew's Hospital in London explained to his students that "[t]here is but one way to obtain knowledge ... we must be companions with the dead."[3] Abernethy was not the only medical professional with this opinion. The London surgeon Sir Astley Cooper encouraged doctors to examine corpses that had died from different diseases. He believed that this practice gave them the opportunity to learn about the progression of a disease without having to perform the same examinations on a living person.[4]

One of the most prolific anatomists of the eighteenth century, William Hunter (1718–1783), also agreed with this mentality. His passion for anatomy allowed him to expand his skills into surgery and obstetrics. During his lifetime he was a member of the Royal Society, in both London and Paris, and a member of the Society of Antiquaries. By 1746, Hunter had begun lecturing on anatomy in London. For nearly 20 years (1764–1783), he served as the Physician Extraordinary to Queen Charlotte (the wife of King George III). His findings contributed to multiple areas of medicine and surgery including morbid anatomy, cardiology, and furthering scholarship on the gravid uterus. He was also a strong proponent of the use of cadavers in anatomical studies. Like many respected medical professionals before him, W. Hunter's dissections traversed between both animals and humans, which he preserved and displayed for future study. After he had finished with his own studies on certain dead bodies, he also preserved and displayed them for future scholars to study. He believed that the skills necessary to display and preserve the body, such as embalming, boiling, macerating, corroding, injecting, and distilling also fell under the auspices of dissection.[5]

Studying dead bodies was one thing. Getting them was quite another. Despite what happened to Vesalius, people were not regularly donating their family's dead bodies to science. Since it was not actually legal for resurrectionists to disinter corpses, the only legal way to obtain bodies was from the gallows. Until 1752 the number of bodies available was extremely limited. A review of the Bills of Mortality from 1700 to 1758 revealed that only 834 people had been executed for murder during that 58-year period. If the executions that occurred during all of those years were equal, that would allow the medical community to use an average of 14 bodies per year. That, coupled with the growing popularity of medical schools and the general study of medicine, meant that the number of cadavers supplied legally did not meet the amount demanded. After 1752, the legislation changed to allow a nearly limitless number of executed felons to be donated to the Company of Surgeons for dissection. However, not every criminal was executed, and not every practitioner who needed cadavers was a surgeon. So even this did not fulfill the need for cadavers. This meant that the medical community needed to turn to alternative sources, such as graveyards and those who transacted in the illegal but highly necessary commodity of the corpse.

The case of W. Hunter suggests approximately how many bodies were needed by a single teaching professor. He impressed upon his students the importance of using cadavers during their medical education. Hunter's staunch support of the use of several cadavers per lecture came from his own experiences. Throughout his years of study, he attended several anatomy lectures throughout Western Europe, most of which only allowed for one or two corpses, total. He found that this impeded his ability to apply the information that he was learning because there was no direct correlation between the lecture and observing the body. When he began to lecture, he used "a number of dead bodies for one course," in order to allow students to observe body parts in various stages of health.[6] Some of his cadavers may have been affected by disease or infection, by old age, or may have been killed by an accident. When the cadavers had unhealthy body parts, such as those affected by gangrene, rickets, or scurvy, students would have the opportunity to observe them in various stages of disease progression. Since professors like William Hunter took this stance on the use of multiple cadavers, school administers had to get the requisite number of cadavers somehow. If they did not, students could withdraw from those courses, and look for ones that favored hands-on learning over theoretical discussion.

W. Hunter explained that any corpse used for anatomical studies would need to be less than a week old to still be viable. In his opinion, any corpse that was over eight to ten days old would be "of little use."[7] Regarding the viability of the corpse, he explained that "every hour that it is kept, it is losing something of its fitness for anatomical demonstrations."[8] Over his lifetime, Hunter increased the number of lectures he gave in his courses capping at nearly 100 lectures per three month course during the early 1780s. Six cadavers were used in each course.[9] He was so passionate about teaching the study of anatomy that he literally worked himself to death. In 1783, he collapsed while teaching a lecture and died ten days later. Despite his support and usage of cadavers for his courses, he specifically requested not to be dissected after he died.[10]

William Hunter's brother, John, also had an impact on the eighteenth-century medical community. Surgery was still considered to be inferior to medicine. In fact, up until the mid-eighteenth century, most surgical theory was still reliant on the work of Ambroise Paré. This meant that most surgeons functioned as anatomical technicians that primarily focused on limbs and surface wounds. If an infection had settled into a limb, the surgeon had to amputate the limb. Surgeons did not regularly perform surgeries on internal organs. The practice of doing so did not become an expected function of the surgeon until the mid-nineteenth century when antiseptics began to be used to decrease infections. However, J. Hunter believed that there was more to the study of surgery than cutting the body apart. By correlating physiology with surgical procedures, he normalized the study of pathology on diseased limbs.[11]

Like his brother, J. Hunter needed cadavers for his surgical studies. His passion for understanding the human body inspired him to dissect thousands of bodies throughout his career.[12] By doing so, he understood what lay beneath the skin and how the musculature attached to the bones. He understood how the muscles, tissue, and blood vessels worked and how they responded to his invasion of the body. In 1776, J. Hunter was sought out by John Fothergill for assistance with an autopsy on a man who had died suddenly while suffering from angina pectoris during an angry outburst. Through careful examination of the autopsy results, they were able to confirm the connection between angina pectoris and heart disease. In addition, they were able to identify the likelihood that "an occluded coronary artery [w]as the precise seat of the disease."[13]

The tenuous divide between anatomists and surgeons was still in existence. Therefore, unlike the robust education given to medical students, the average surgical student was only taught the basics of anatomy. Having the distinct benefit of being the brother of William Hunter meant that John had spent twelve years learning the study of anatomy before focusing on surgery. This gave him a better foundation to consider the body as a whole being, rather than only focusing on specific parts of the body and how they would be affected by surgery.

Had John Hunter's impact on Enlightenment medicine ended with surgery, it would have been quite enough. His understanding of anatomy worked in his favor, and he became a highly sought London surgeon. He approached surgery methodically and believed that every action performed on the body should have a specific purpose. His thought process was based in science, and he took the act of practicing surgery seriously. However, despite his enlightened mindset, his career took an alternate path. Rather than remaining in the academic system as a surgeon and scholar, he chose to go down the path of resurrectionism.

In 1798, there were approximately 300 anatomy students studying in London.[14] By 1823, that number had increased to nearly 1,000, although it did decrease to approximately 800 by 1828.[15] Of the 800 anatomy students studying in London, only about 500 of them needed cadavers for their dissections, each of which needed at least three cadavers throughout the sixteen-month program. This meant that a minimum of 1,500 cadavers were needed per program, for students alone. Since it was not possible for the medical community to obtain enough cadavers though legal means, they were forced to buy cadavers from resurrectionists in order to keep up with the demand. However, some people received more than they bargained for when it was discovered that the bodies that they had purchased were still very much alive.

Such was the case for John Macintyre, who had the unfortunate experience of being proclaimed as dead, was buried, and woke up on the autopsy table in 1824. Alarmingly, Macintyre recalled the journey to and from the grave. After losing the ability to move, he heard the nurse proclaim him to be dead. He recalled that after a time, he was placed into his coffin and then the coffin was lowered into the grave. Although not fully conscious, he was keenly aware that dirt was being shoveled on top of his coffin. Certain that he would die, he was hopeful when he heard the dirt above him moving again. He had hoped that it was his friends coming to dig him out. Instead resurrectionists wielded the shovel. After pulling him out of the grave, they brought him to a local medical school. Macintyre recounted the following testimonial of his awakening:

> Being rudely stripped of my shroud, I was placed naked on a table. In a short time I heard by the bustle in the room that the doctors and students were assembling. When all was ready the Demonstrator took his knife, and pierced my bosom. I felt a dreadful crackling, as it were, throughout my whole frame; a convulsive shudder instantly followed, and a shriek of horror rose from all present. The ice of death was broken up; my trance was ended. The utmost exertions were made to restore me, and in the course of an hour I was in full possession of all my faculties.[16]

Rumors circulated about others who were misdiagnosed as dead and returned to life when grave robbers tried to steal valuables out their tomb or coffin. The following story was reported to Dr. William Hawes—a well-respected physician and medical administrator in eighteenth-century London. Hawes then included it in the 1787 report of the Royal Humane Society: the mother of a lady who lived in Hertfordshire was brought back "to life after interment by the attempt of a thief to steal a valuable ring from her finger."[17] Despite the simplistic storyline, the retelling included elements of truth. Primary sources from the time used the words "premature burial" to designate people who had been buried in the ground after they had been incorrectly diagnosed as dead and "premature interment" to explain those who had been interred into a vault after the same misdiagnosis had been made. Vault burials were much more expensive and could only be afforded by the rich. If the lady had been of a respectable lineage, her mother would have been interred in the family tomb. The grave robbers in this story had been interested in stealing the jewels that the woman was buried with, rather than the corpse of the woman herself. In a way, she was lucky that they had broken into her vault and tried to take her ring. She may not have woken up otherwise. Or, when she did awaken, she would have been trapped with no way to escape. Since it is plausible that corpses were coming back to life when grave robbers were disturbing the grave, it is possible that they were doing so when resurrectionists were disturbing the body in a tomb or vault. Three of the sketches presented in the *Uncertainty and Signs of Death* (1746) depicted people coming back to life when a resurrectionist opened the coffin. One picture depicts the opening of a coffin inside a mausoleum or tomb. The person who opened it received quite a surprise when the person inside sat up, alive.

* * *

Despite the commonality of resurrectionists there were other laws in place to try to provide the medical community with enough cadavers. In 1625, the scholar and statesmen Hugo Grotius indicated the right to be properly buried could be withheld from the worst of criminals because their bodies were considered to be property of the state. This premise coupled with allowances like those set forth by King Henry VIII, Elizabeth I, and King Charles II made gathering bodies from the scaffolds for anatomical use a normality in England.

There were times when the Royal College of Physicians paid people to collect bodies from executions and bring them back to the College for anatomical study. Concerns for the sanctity of the soul and respect for the remains of the body dictated that the RCP would be responsible for the proper burial of those bodies. As per a decree made by the President of the Royal College of Physicians, Charles Goodall, in 1709, the bodies that were taken from the gallows and used by the College were to be "decently buried at the cost and Charges of the said Profit Colleges or Community."[18] The burial of those who had committed crimes against oneself, such as self-murder (suicide) or felonious acts against others were handled differently than burials of those who had lived virtuous lives and died of natural causes. Neither Catholic nor Protestants allowed for the bodies of those who had killed themselves to be buried in a churchyard, unless a coroner's jury had concluded that the death was due to insanity.[19] Likewise, those bodies could not be dissected. The death historian Thomas Laqueur explained that the "refusal to properly bury a corpse … constituted a posthumous exclusion from the cultural and political order, an obliteration of personhood after death."[20] This was why, after criminals had been executed at the gallows, their bodies could be given to medical professionals for academic study or, later, to surgeons for public dissection.

Proof of post-dissection burials were discovered when the Museum of London Archeology (MOLA) excavated Royal London Hospital's graveyard in 2006. They found that 144 of the 273 excavated graves contained portions of bodies from an estimated 500 individuals.[21] These body parts were predominantly from men, but the remains of women, children, and fetuses were also discovered. The remains showed signs of dissection, such as "craniotomies, vertebral transition at the neck or lumbar spine, … pelvic hemisection … and thoracotomies."[22] Ann Millard, the wife of a resurrectionist, wrote detailed accounts of her husband, William disinterring corpses from the Royal London Hospital Burial ground during the 1820s.

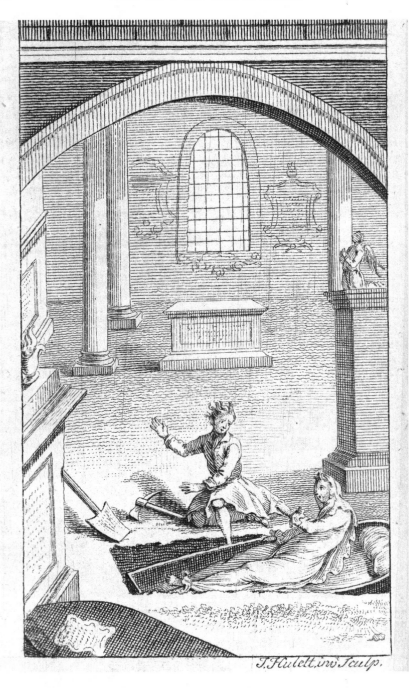

A grave robber or resurrectionist gets surprised when the person he uncovers is alive (used with permission from the Wellcome Collection).

The bodies were sold back to Royal London Hospital as well as other to other interested anatomists. Ironically, William Millard was imprisoned in Coldbath Fields prison after being "apprehended in the London Hospital burial ground in dubious circumstance" and later died there.[23]

In order to increase the number of corpses legally available to the medical community, the number of bodies that were allowed to be used for anatomical dissections increased again in 1752. King George II approved legislation named the "Act for Better Preventing the Horrid Crime of Murder" (25 Geo. 2.c.37), which was commonly referred to as the Murder Act. This legislation allowed for the executed bodies of all murders to be used by the Company of Surgeons, or their designee, for medical dissections.[24] Judges were given the option of sentencing the criminal to have their body dissected either privately or publicly after the execution.[25] After the body was granted to the Company of Surgeons, it was not allowed to be buried until it had been dissected. If the person had been sentenced to be dissected by anatomists, the body would be privately dissected, and the information obtained would be used for academic study. Conversely, if the person had been sentenced to be publicly dissected, the body would be dissected in front of others and examined in great detail in order to validate that the person had died during the execution.

The Murder Act was created as a deterrent to committing murder. It worked. Those of the working and poor classes in England responded with fear for their immortal souls. The educated jurors, however, recognized the extreme nature and long-term, religious ramifications of the law and used it sparingly. Between 1752 and 1832, only 923 bodies of convicts were brought before the court, executed, and sentenced to postmortem dissection.[26] As observed between 1700 and 1758, this legislation did not supply enough cadavers for the physicians, surgeons, anatomists, and students within London's medical community.

This left anatomists, surgeons, and their students in quite a bind. The number of corpses needed for dissection rose in correlation with the increased number of students entering medical school. At a time before x-rays or even photographs, hands-on invasive dissections of the body was the best way to learn about the anatomy and physiology and how the bodily systems functioned in conjunction with each other, or were affected by injury or disease. Resurrectionists continued to be used to fill in the gap between what the medical community needed and what the legal system could supply.

The blending of morality and legality during the eighteenth century was evident by how the two concepts were linked together when it came to the laws regulating the corpse. Possibly due to the work that the medical community had done to delineate the differences between life and death, the corpse was no longer viewed as a person. In addition, there was a divide between the national and local administrations because "national issues often did not interest townsfolk as much as the need to solve the various local problems."[27] In response, the regulations regarding the theft of the corpse were eased and the consequence of doing so was reduced from a felony to a misdemeanor in 1788. This shift in the law created a loophole that made it easier for corpses to be disinterred by resurrectionists. This decision came with its own societal concerns. People were still concerned about the fate of their souls. Therefore, there were still concerns that the physical separation of the body would hinder the ability for soul to find the body in order to be reunited during the Reckoning.

The acceptance of the role of the resurrectionist increased throughout the eighteenth century and laws were created to protect and govern the process. In 1788, it was decided that civil action could not be taken against someone who violated or disturbed the actual remains of a corpse, as long as the body was being removed to further "the improvement of the science of anatomy."[28] This legislation came as an outcome of the *Rex v Lynn* case (*Rex* v. *Lynn, M. 1788, 2 T.R. 733*), which reduced the consequences of exhuming the body from the felony of theft to a misdemeanor of "public indecency."[29] Since the corpse no longer held the essence of life, it did not fall under the auspice of kidnapping. The burial of the corpse indicated that family had abandoned it, so it was managed by the "abandoned property" laws. Although it was legally acceptable for the resurrectionist to remove the body from the ground, that was all that they could remove. The coffin, winding sheet, burial shroud, or personal belongings that were buried with the person were still considered to be the property of the family. Therefore, taking those items would fall under the charge of felonious theft.

In 1786, the *Ipswich Journal* published this story depicting the theft of a body and the articles buried with it.

> About 12 o'clock at night, Mr. Tankard and his man coming by the churchyard, observed some men a digging, and a cart standing by, they watched the motion of those *resurrection* men, and presently saw them open the coffin and take out the *body*, which consisted of upwards of 500 pieces of muslin, and various other contraband articles. Mr. Tankard suffered them to proceed with the *corpse* till they came to Ratcliffe-cross, where he got assistance, and seized the whole.[30]

Since this story took place prior to the *Rex v. Lynn* case, the theft of the body was considered to be a felony and the items taken were considered immaterial. However, if it had taken place a few years later, the removal of the body would have been a misdemeanor and the taking the items out of the coffin would have been considered theft.

Resurrectionists had a hierarchy within their ranks. Those who had made successful connections within the medical community would sometimes hire others to perform the labor of digging up the body. Due to their not quite legal status, resurrectionists tended to work at night, often bribing the guard of local cemeteries and graveyards to either turn a blind eye or even assist if the price was right. It can be assumed that digging dirt out of the grave, as well as breaking coffins open or removing them from the burial plot would make a considerable amount of noise. This commotion would be ignored by those that they paid off, making it easier to abscond with the dead weight of a body. When disinterring a body, the goal was two-fold: (1) extraction of the body and (2) make sure that it looked like they had never been there.

Only the first of these goals were met in the textual evidence provided in legal paperwork regarding a case of "body stealing" which had occurred in Yaxley, England. In November 1830, a London resurrectionist by the name of "Grimmer" connected with a man named William Patrick, who lived approximately 80 miles away in Farcet, which is situated between Yaxley and Peterborough, England. Grimmer offered Patrick the opportunity to "raise [me] a dead body or two."[31] After Patrick agreed to do so, Grimmer instructed him to dig up the corpse of Jane Mason who had been recently buried in the Yaxley Churchyard. After gaining permission from Grimmer, Patrick asked his friend William Whayley to assist him since Whayley had previously assisted him in digging up another body.

Whayley, initially, denied the opportunity to assist, even after being offered a sovereign as payment. But Patrick was persistent. After a night of drinking together, Patrick handed his friend a sack and gathered tools such as a plankhook and a shovel. They walked to the Yaxley Churchyard, where Patrick shoveled the dirt out of the grave and cleared off the coffin. After unscrewing the part of the coffin lid that covered the head and shoulders, Patrick instructed Whayley to hold back the coffin lid. Whayley did as asked, at which time Patrick slid Jane's body out of the coffin and put it in the sack. Her clothes were removed and put back in the grave, at which point the dirt was replaced on top of the coffin.

While they were taking the body back to Farcet, Patrick shared that he hoped to become the middleman within the year, because that was who made the most money. He considered the middleman to be the person who connected with the medical professionals who needed the body and was not the person responsible for disinterring it. Since it was getting late, they decided to put Mason's corpse in a ditch, and Patrick would return for it in the morning. But by the time he returned, the body had been found and taken away to a local alehouse for safe keeping until it could be identified. One of the people called in to try to identify the body, a man named

Billings, recognized the body as his recently deceased wife. In order to assuage any concerns about the body being incorrectly identified, he went to check his wife's grave. Upon return, he reported that her body was missing from her grave at the Peterborough Burial Ground. He brought her empty coffin back to the alehouse and Jane was put inside. The coffin was closed up and Jane was interred in Mrs. Billings' grave at Peterborough Burial Ground.

It did not take long for Patrick to find out what happened to the body. When Grimmer returned to pick up the corpse of Jane Mason, he was informed about the mishandling of the body and where it was currently buried. The two of them rode in Grimmer's cart to the Peterborough Burial Ground, and together they re-disinterred the body. They loaded Jane's body into Grimmer's cart and parted company.[32] It is not known if Patrick ever became a middleman.

Societal allowances, like those seen in the Farcet story, made it easier for resurrectionists to exhume freshly buried bodies. As seen in this story, people were so comfortable with the concept of digging up a grave that they would do it themselves in order to check on their loved ones. In 1795, a company of 15 resurrectionists who worked out of the London borough of Lambeth was exposed to the public. They worked during the winter because the cold helped preserve the bodies and sold their commodity to eight reputable (but unnamed) surgeons. Other companies exhumed bodies from hospital graveyards and then sold the bodies back to medical professionals.[33] It was rumored that the more seasoned resurrectionists could remove two bodies from different graves in less than an hour and a half, including placing the coffins back in the grave and filling the hole.[34]

Another company of resurrectionists stole bodies from the burial ground associated with the pesthouse that used to be located on Old Street Road, London. Upon noticing that a hackney coach was parked nearby, "the parish watchmen were ordered to keep a good look out."[35] When one of the watchmen approached the coach, "he was assaulted and beaten by three men, who then made off."[36] The coachman was taken into custody, at which time it was noticed that there were three sacks in his coach; two held one man's body each and the third held the bodies of three children. When the burial ground was searched, several more bodies were located underneath the outer wall; they looked like they had been set there to be carried off later. It was "generally believed, that almost all the bodies deposited there for five weeks past have been stole, which, upon an average, must have been about fifteen per week."[37] The coachman reported that he was supposed to have been paid ten guineas for his service that night. Instead, he was sent to New Prison in Clerkenwell, London and was locked up with the bodies that were found in his coach. After sleeping so soundly that he was difficult to awaken, he was brought before the Magistrate the next day. Unfortunately, as with many of the reports of the time, no follow-up was published regarding what ultimately happened to the coachman.

Techniques used by resurrectionists to remove the body from its grave without being caught were considered to be a mystery to those outside of the trade, even during the eighteenth century. B.B. Cooper claimed that Sir Astley had asked one of his contacts in the resurrectionist community about their trade secrets. He was informed that one of the most important things to do was to pay the cemetery watchmen. This payoff was so common that the family and friends of the deceased would sometimes hire people to stand watch over their graves until the body would have lost its freshness. If they could not afford to hire someone, sometimes they would stand watch themselves. One of the larger hospitals in London had a burial ground adjacent to it. This area was used to bury the bodies of those who had been dissected. Ironically, the hospital administers were concerned about the safety of the dissected corpses that were buried there. In order to keep their burial ground safe, they employed a well-known and adept resurrectionist as the watchman. They paid him well so that he would not be able to be bribed by other resurrectionists. The time came when another resurrectionist was employed by a surgeon from that same hospital to exhume a body that had been recently buried there. Although the new guard could not be bribed, he glutted himself so thoroughly with his dinner and drink that he fell to sleep at his post. This allowed the other resurrectionist to disinter the requested body and deliver it to the surgeon of the hospital.

In addition to maintaining unscrupulous connections with the cemetery watchmen, resurrectionists made quick, stealthy work of disinterring their preferred body. A skilled resurrectionist could work so quickly and quietly that they were able to get their preferred corpse while a guard went for dinner or took a nap. Echoing the body stealing case from Farcet, B.B. Cooper shared the following method of releasing a corpse from its coffin. Dirt would be cleared from about ⅓ of the coffin lid, from the chest area to the head. A crow-bar would be forced into the space between the lid and the bottom of the coffin. By using the crowbar as a lever, it was easy to pry the lid open. Since the rest of the coffin lid was weighed down by dirt, the weight bearing upon the coffin lid would often cause the lid to break. After this, the body would be slid out of the coffin, and any clothing, shrouds, cloth, and/or belongings removed and placed back into the coffin. The body was then "tied up and placed in its receptacle to be conveyed to its destination."[38] Finally, the dirt was replaced into the grave.

In order to keep up with the demand, resurrectionists often had to exhume multiple bodies in a night, sometimes during one dig. This technique was especially useful when various disease outbreaks killed large quantities of people at a time. In these cases, coffins were often buried stacked three or four high and not buried very deeply. In order to obtain as many bodies as possible the earth above and around the coffin would be removed. Since the coffins were stacked, it was easier to pull them out in succession, remove the body, and then replace them back in their original order before the grave was filled in with dirt.[39]

Another description of the tactics used to extract bodies from graves was published in the December 9, 1817, issue of the *Hull Packet*. In this case, Mr. Seager, the sexton of a parish in Lambeth, interrupted the resurrectionists at work:

> On Sunday night they concealed them-selves in a convenient part of the burial-ground, and about ten o'clock observed two men passing over the graves. They first proceeded to that part of the ground where there were two man-traps set, which they let off; they then proceeded to the bone house, broke it open, and provided themselves with spades, and immediately afterwards commenced their operations upon a grave wherein a body had been deposited the preceding day. Mr. Seager continued to watch their proceedings; they dug till the spades struck a coffin. Mr. Seager then came from his concealment, and called out to these men to desist and surrender themselves; then discovered to his great astonishment, that they were the identical persons whom he had hired and paid to protect the ground.[40]

Another trick of the trade was how the resurrectionists moved the bodies from the grave to the hospital, school, or medical professional. Often, the body would be transferred by cart or coach. The October 15, 1819, issue of the *Public Ledger and Daily Advertiser* discussed a case where people were caught transporting a body to the Brompton section of London:

> The hamper and matted bundle, containing the bodies, were brought by a man and a soldier to Brompton, where they were placed on the roof of the coach. The man who applied for the parcels at the Inn was brought forward; he was recognized by a Constable of East Grinstead to have been formerly a carrier of that place, but subsequently obtained his living by procuring subjects for Surgeons.[41]

Not only did resurrectionists face legal ramifications for their actions, but the medical professionals that used the bodies purchased from the resurrectionists did as well. Anyone who received the disinterred bodies was "liable to be tried for a misdemeanor, with a risk of incurring severe penalties."[42] Whether they knew, or cared, was of little difference, however. The bodies were needed, so professors, doctors, surgeons, and hospital or medical school administrators, worked out of back doors and made discrete deals to procure the bodies that they needed for their students and to advance the study of medicine.

The poem "Mary's Ghost," initially published in Thomas Hood's *Whims and Oddities* (1826), used dry wit to explain the role of the resurrectionist and medical practitioners. The poem was narrated by the deceased Mary to her significant other Thomas and used popular imagery to reflect her perspective as her body parts were bought and sold to different medical facilities and practitioners around London. This was the sort of physical separation of the body that had so many worried about the soul finding its body and both being able to reanimate during the Reckoning. The poem began by lamenting her plight:

> I thought the last of all my cares
> Would end with my last minute;
> But, tho' I went to my long home,
> I didn't stay long in it.
>
> The body-snatchers they have come,
> And made a snatch at me;
> It's very hard them kind of men
> Won't let a body be!
>
> You thought that I was buried deep
> Quite decent like and chary,
> But from her grace in Mary-bone
> They've come and boned your Mary[43] [v3–5].

The following verse mentioned Sir Astley as one of the practitioners who received a piece of her body. Then the poem concluded by explaining how little of her body remains in its grave.

> The cock it crows—I must be gone!
> My William, we must part!
> But, I'll be yours in death, altho'
> Sir Astley has my heart.
>
> Don't go to weep upon my grave,
> And think that there I be;
> They haven't left an atom there
> Of my anatomie [*sic*][44] [v11–12].

Hood was not the only poet to use the underbelly of the early modern medicine as the macabre plotline for poetry from the same era. At the end of the eighteenth century, Robert Southey wrote at length in his verse *The Surgeon's Warning* (1798). The poem was narrated by a surgeon who mused at the end of his life about what would happen to his body after he died. In a poetic echo of what may have been considered by W. Hunter towards the end of his life, Southey's fictionalized surgeon described the actions that had been taken against other bodies and the awareness that his death would leave his own body vulnerable to the same actions.

Initially, the narrator requested that the parson and undertaker come to his side because his death was imminent. However, the news of his near demise brought his apprentices to his side. Despite being their teacher, he was not happy to see them—or the resurrectionist that snuck in with them—and sent them away. He mentioned that he had worked with Joseph, called "Mister Joe" later in the poem.

The Parson and the Undertaker

They hastily came complying,
And the Surgeon's Prentices ran up stairs
When they heard that their Master was dying.

The Prentices all they enter'd the room,
By one, by two, by three;
With a sly grin came Joseph in
First of the company.

The Surgeon swore as they enter'd his door,
'T was fearful his oaths to hear,...
"Now send these scoundrels out of my sight,
I beseech ye, my brethren dear!"[45] [v3–5].

In both cases—when referring to his apprentices and the resurrectionist—he was concerned that they would act in accordance with their roles in the medical community. He feared that the "rascal Joe would be at [him]" after he died but did not want to see him before that time had come. He lamented about how his apprentices would "surely come and carve me bone from bone."[46] He admitted to the irony that he "who have rifled the dead man's grave shall never have rest in my own."[47] The narrator even went so far as to admit what had done to "rifle" through other people's graves. He worked with both resurrectionists and church sexton and "cut up" their bodies in order to make tallow candles of human fat and dried bodies and organs in order to preserve them for study.[48]

The surgeon narrator also made requests regarding what he wanted to happen to his body in order to keep his apprentices and the resurrectionists from exhuming, dissecting, or studying it. He asked to be buried in a lead coffin with the top soldered closed and then to have the coffin weighed to ensure that he was inside. Then, he asked that the lead coffin be put inside another coffin. He hoped that this would protect his body if the outer coffin got stolen or opened, because his body would still be protected and the lead coffin would be difficult to break into. Then he requested that his double enclosed body be buried inside his brother's church and the key well-guarded. Had his been biographical, rather than a poem that reflected the concerns of the time, the request to be buried in his brother's church would have indicated that his brother was a man of stature because only the rich and powerful could be buried inside of a church. Otherwise, he would have been buried in outside in the cemetery with everyone else.

After being encased in two coffins and buried inside a locked church, he also asked that three large men guard his grave inside the church for three weeks. Payment included alcohol, a blunderbuss and ammunition, and the promise of additional money if they shot a resurrectionist. After the three week period he believed that his body would have decayed enough to be worthless to the resurrectionist or his apprentices.

> And all night long let three stout men
> The vestry watch within;
> To each man give a gallon of beer,
> And a keg of Holland's gin;
>
> Powder and ball and blunderbuss,
> To save me if he can,
> And eke five guineas if he shoot
> A Resurrection Man[49] [v15–16].

Unfortunately, for the narrator, the sexton of the church was already working with the resurrectionist, Mr. Joe. Night after night, the sexton came in with an offering of more and more money until at last he offered the guards three guineas for permission to take the body. After the guards agreed to sell the body that they were hired to protect, the sexton let Mr. Joe in so that the surgeon's body could be disinterred. They broke the floor with pick-axes and then shoveled through the clay that had been laid on top of the coffin. They broke open the outer coffin and then the inner one and put the surgeon in sack to be carried away and sold.

The poem ends with an explanation about the stench of the rotting corpse that was so foul that it could be smelled by the guards who passed from about twelve feet away. This meant that the final corpse was likely too old to be useful and the resurrectionists were unlikely to sell the body because it had degraded beyond its point of usability.

* * *

The business of the corpse as a commodity continued to grow throughout the early nineteenth century, finally coming to a head in 1828. The public were becoming more aware of the resurrectionist's actions and started to come up with different ways to protect the corpse. In some cases, cages, called mortsafes, were erected over graves in order to keep resurrectionists out and the body inside. As obtaining corpses became more difficult, the price that resurrectionists charged the medical community increased. In 1800 the average price of a corpse was one to two guineas, which would have the approximate purchase power of £85—£171 in 2020. By 1828, the cost had increased to 10 guineas for an adult corpse (approximately £1,168 in 2020) and 16 guineas for an adult corpse with anatomical differences (approximately £1,862 in 2020).[50]

Also in 1828, a Select Committee was created in the House of Commons to discuss how medical schools obtained cadavers. After hearing evidence from "distinguished members of the medical profession, a number of magistrates, and three unnamed resurrectionists," the Committee compared the increased need for cadavers for medical training against the limitations of their current laws.[51] In order to supplement the amount of bodies legally supplied they recommended that the bodies of people who were "maintained at the public charge" and who were unclaimed after they died in "charitable institutions," such as workhouses, penitentiaries, prisons, and hospitals, be turned over to the anatomists for dissection.[52] The Committee reviewed the number of people who had died at the St. Giles in the Field workhouse (London) in 1827–1828. They determined that of the 585 people who had died and been buried at the expense of the parish, 20 percent, or 117, were unclaimed. Turning the bodies over to anatomists was considered to be a win-win scenario. Medical professionals would get the bodies that they needed for their studies. Meanwhile, parishes would save money on burials because the medical professionals would be responsible for burying the remains of the body after the dissection. The bill was drafted with the support of the Select Committee. However, the motion was withdrawn because provisions could not be assured for a "Christian burial" to take place for the post-dissection remains.[53]

As the Committee discussed and debated how to change the laws relating to cadavers, some resurrectionists in Scotland took things to the next level. Casually termed "burking," a small number of resurrectionists in England and Scotland killed people in order to sell the freshest corpses that money could buy. Arguably, two of the most famous burkers in the history of medicine were the Scottish body snatchers Burke and Hare. In 1828, William Burke and William Hare were convicted of murder in order to supply Dr. Robert Knox with fresh corpses for his anatomical dissections. Burke and Hare preyed on the most vulnerable of living society. Mostly, they focused their efforts on murdering the poor, homeless, orphans, or those with intellectual disabilities. Over the course of a year, "they provided 16 bodies for Dr. Knox's anatomy class."[54] Their serial murdering ways came to an end, however, after they murdered Madgy Docherty on October 31, 1828. Rather than delivering her body directly to Knox, they hid it in the lodge house where they lived. Unfortunately for them, a neighbor took notice of the body and alerted the authorities.

When they were questioned about the murders, Hare turned on Burke and disappeared into history. Burke was found guilty and hung for the crime of murder. As part of his sentence, he was publicly dissected. The purpose of his dissection being public was to shame him, even after death—his insides laying open for all in attendance to see. Dr. Knox was implicated in these murders as his supply chain fell apart. He claimed not to have knowledge of how Burke and Hare obtained the corpses that they sold to him. Despite his protestations, his reputation had been tarnished and it took years for him to repair it. Since his death, his name has been irrevocably attached to Burke, Hare, and the murders that illuminated one of the darkest shadows of the advancement of medicine in the early modern era.

As though murdering for the sake of monetary gain was not deplorable enough, Scotland's Burke and Hare murders resulted in copycats in England. The intrinsic link between the medical community and the resurrectionists had been acceptable for nearly a century. Who medical practitioners and administrators worked with was almost as important as the state of the body when it was delivered. W. Hunter had taught about the importance of receiving fresh bodies in his anatomy classes. However, there was a difference in decay between a body that had died, been watched, and been buried, and a body that been killed and delivered directly afterwards. This became an issue on Saturday, November 5, 1831, when the resurrectionists, John Bishop and James May, brought the abnormally fresh body of a young boy, to William Hill, the porter of Kings College London. They told Hill that the boy was fourteen years old and asked for a price of 12 guineas. Hill went and got the demonstrator of Anatomy at the college, Richard Partridge. Partridge was able to negotiate the price down to nine guineas. After agreeing upon the price, they took the body out of their sack and mentioned that "the body was fresh."[55]

Upon seeing the body, Hill asked how the boy had died. He received the reply "It was no business of theirs, nor his."[56] Hill noticed that the boy's body was not in a position indicative of having been prepared for burial and discussed his concerns with Partridge. Partridge noticed that the boy had sustained several injuries, such as a cut to the left temple, that his lips and face were swollen, his eyes were bloodshot, and his limbs rigid. In addition to the boy's injuries, he noticed that the body was exceptionally fresh. Concerned that the boy met an untimely demise through violent means, Partridge excused himself to get money in order to pay for the body. Instead of doing so, he went to the police and then stopped by the Secretary's office on his way back to pick up a £50 note before returning to the group. When Partridge returned to the room, he noticed that Thomas Williams, another resurrectionist who had been working in the hospital, had joined the Bishop and May. Partridge explained that he did not have the exact amount of money for the body. The resurrectionists discussed taking a partial payment at the time, and Bishop offered to come back on Monday for the rest of the payment. May offered to take the note and get it changed out. Partridge turned down both offers. Soon after, the police arrived and Bishop, May, and Williams, plus the fourth resurrectionist in their group, named Michael Shields, were taken into custody. The boy's body was taken to the Covent Garden Police Station and placed in the custody of the Superintendent of Police, Mr. Thomas. The following day Partridge went to the police station to properly examine the body.

Vagrancy was a problem in London during the mid-nineteenth century. It was estimated that there were 15,000 vagrant children living in London during the late 1820s.[57] These children often performed as street entertainers or walking marketers for tradesmen, although some did turn to unofficial trades such as theft and pickpocketing. Some showed off animals, such as monkeys, white mice, porcupines, or dancing dogs to passers-by for a modest fee. Many of these children had been living in Italy when they were sold into a child trafficking ring. Their parents made deals with people called padroni or padrones, who were loosely responsible for overseeing the child. These padroni would pay the parents for their children and would promise that they would teach the children a trade. The trade was generally expected to be some form of performance or theater. Instead, the children were brought to England and taught how to busk for alms. Known as the "Italian Boy" trade, this child-trafficking ring extended across England, those who were brought to London boarded in and around Holborn and on the south end of Drury Lane.

The boy was identified as Carlo Ferrari, also known as Charles Ferrier. During the trial of the Williams, Bishop, and May, the British press dubbed Carlo Ferrari "The Italian Boy." Carlo's particular trade was animal exhibitions, and he was often seen with a little cage hanging from his neck which he used to show off a tortoise or white mice running on a wheel. He lodged at "Mr. Elliott's," at 2 Charles Street, on Drury Lane in London. Carlo came to England two years earlier, under the "guardianship" of the padrone Augustine Brun.[58] During the trial, Brun admitted that he had brought Carlo from Italy and that the last time he had seen him alive was on July 28, 1830.

According to a report of the trial, published in the *London Courier and Evening Gazette* on December 2, 1831, closer observation of the outside of Carlo's corpse did not reveal any evidence of foul play, and the cut along the left temple was not deep. However, Carlo's teeth had been removed, his jaw and gums were broken, and blood remained on his gums. There was a wound on the back of the head, which seemed to indicate that it had been struck soundly while he had been living. Upon opening the body,

Partridge observed that the chest, abdomen, stomach, spinal cord, and brain were in good condition. As he began to look deeper, however, he found that blood had coagulated in the membrane that surrounds the spinal cord, in the spinal canal, and in the corresponding muscles at the back of the neck. It was concluded that Carlo had died from receiving "blows sufficient to cause death."[59] Partridge explained that the swelling of the lips and face and the bloodshot eyes were also symptoms of such a death. When questioned about the health of the heart, he explained that the lack of blood in the heart meant that Carlo had died suddenly. It was a cold November, so the state of the body indicated that Carlo had been dead for less than 36 hours. It was also determined that the body had never been laid out to be watched, since the lack of sawdust in his hair indicated that he had never been in a coffin.

John Bishop, James May, and Michael Shields had all been well-known resurrectionists in London. Bishop, May, and Williams were arrested for the murder of Carlo Ferrari. This particular case was considered to be different than typical resurrectionism because "the prisoners stood charged with the murder of a poor boy, for the purpose of possessing themselves of the dead body, that they might obtain money for it by disposing of it to the surgeons for dissection."[60] That said, there was a general feeling that if the investigation had resulted in evidence that created a reasonable amount of doubt, then the jury would "give the prisoners the full benefit of such a feeling."[61] John Bishop had been unapologetically a part of the resurrectionist trade for over a decade and already served time in jail for it. James May had been involved in the trade for approximately six years and had been arrested and convicted for grave-robbing.[62] However, he was adamant that he had never taken "undue advantage of any person alive, whether man, woman, or child, however poor or unprotected."[63] Thomas Williams was new to the resurrectionist gang and joined the trade after recently serving time in prison for theft. Michael Shields was only tangently related to the case because he happened to be there when Bishop and May attempted to sell Carlo's body to William Hill at Kings College London; therefore, he acted as a witness and was not put on trial.

The murder indictment for John Bishop and Thomas Williams, and James May was held on December 1, 1831. After a discussion regarding the state of the body and how had been transported to Kings College London, Bishop confessed to murdering Ferrari on November 3, 1831. He claimed that May did not know about the murder. Bishop also admitted to murdering a boy who went by the name of Cunningham on October 21, 1831, and Fanny Pigburn on October 9, 1831. Williams admitted to being an accomplice in these murders but denied having ever had any other experience in burking or resurrectionist activity. He also provided the court with important information about how bodies were moved and which watchmen overlooked resurrectionist activity. In the end, John Bishop, Thomas Williams, and James May were found to be guilty and sentenced to death. The executed bodies of John Bishop and Thomas Williams were dissected by the Royal College of Surgeons in London by the end of the year.

The bond between the resurrectionists and the medical community, which had been imperative for the advancement of medical study in the previous century, now bound them together in public scrutiny. Not only did the public distrust the work habits and morals of the resurrectionists, but they also doubted the medical community at large. In response, Parliament reviewed the points that had been discussed by the Select Committee in 1828. In 1829, the "Bill for Preventing the Unlawful Disinterment of Human Bodies, and for Regulating the Schools of Anatomy" was proposed to the House of Commons. The purpose of this bill was to discourage people from disinterring bodies from cemeteries, burial grounds, or vaults, and to provide licenses for those who performed dissections. A panel of commissioners was to be appointed, provided that the majority of them were not from the medical community. Rather than getting the bodies from the ground, it was proposed that the bodies of those who died in hospitals and workhouses, which had been unclaimed for over 48 hours, would be given to the medical community to continue to support medical advancement. The legislation also allowed for bodies to be legally donated to the medical community for the same purpose. Dissections could occur only in licensed buildings and a license would be needed transport a body. Most importantly, all bodies that were used for anatomical dissections were required to be buried. If this step was skipped, then the medical professional would be fined £50.

The proposed bill was not received well. It was considered to be hateful towards the poor because it made their bodies easily available for dissection. There were also concerns that the poor would not go to workhouses or hospitals if they felt that their bodies were going to be sold to the medical community after they died. Not everyone in the medical community was enthusiastic about it either. Independent teachers and the administrators of small medical schools were concerned that their inability to pay for the proposed licenses would cause them to close when students began to favor the larger medical schools and corporations. The *Lancet* had satirically nicknamed the legislation "A Bill for Preventing Country Surgeons from Studying Anatomy." The bill was so poorly received that even medical associations like the College of Surgeons formed petitions against it.[64] Additional concerns were raised regarding the panel of commissioners overseeing the whole practice of surgery, especially when no one on the commission was expected to be a surgeon.

Instead, the "Act for Regulating the Schools of Anatomy," usually called the Anatomy Act of 1832, was instituted to produce a legal supply of cadavers for the medical community and to grant licenses to those who practiced anatomy. It was also intended to reduce the number of "grievous crimes" that were committed to acquire cadavers.[65] Most importantly, it was intended to allow medical professionals to gain access to an adequate number of cadavers from sources other than resurrectionists. Anyone who practiced anatomy was required to apply for licensure to do so. In order to prove that the applicants were legitimate practitioners of anatomy, the applications needed to be signed by two justices of the peace who were active in the area that the medical practitioner or student taught, practiced, or studied. This new legislation applied to anyone who was "lawfully qualified to practice medicine in any part of the United Kingdom."[66] These qualified practitioners included anyone who had graduated from or had attained a licentiate in medicine, the fellows and members of the Colleges of Physicians and/or Surgeons, professors of anatomy, surgery, or medicine, and all students who were attending school for anatomy. The new legislation also provided for an oversight committee of at least three inspectors. These inspectors would be appointed to oversee the lawful practice of anatomy in towns and communities. They were responsible for reporting the demographical information of the cadavers used for anatomical dissections including name, age, and sex of each corpse.

The "Act for Regulating the Schools of Anatomy" repealed the Murder Act of 1752, thus ending the ability to receive corpses of criminals from the gallows. Instead, it allowed people who had legal custody of a body to "permit the body of such deceased person to undergo anatomical examination," provided that the person with legal custody was not an undertaker or another person entrusted to bury the body.[67] By allowing bodies to be donated in this way, the government had endeavored to provide a never ending supply of free corpses for anatomical study. The processing of this paperwork also provided extra days for the body to show signs of decay, increasing the certainty of death. The rights of the dying person were also taken into consideration. The dying person had the right to request that their body not be turned over to the medical community for dissection. The legislation stipulated that the legal holder of the body could not turn the body over for dissection if

to the knowledge of such executor or other party, such person shall have expressed his desire, either in writing at any time during his life, or verbally in the presence of two or more witnesses during the illness whereof he died that his body after death might not undergo such examination, or unless the surviving husband or wife, or any known relative of the deceased person, shall require the body to be interred without such examination.[68]

Concerns about the state of the soul during and after the time of death and fears of what would happen to the soul should the body be exhumed and/or separated were still valid to many. In these cases, the lawful possession of the body referred to the friends or family who were in possession of the recently deceased. Many times the law was used to validate workhouses that donated the bodies of the dead poor to the medical community. In those cases, the body could be released after 48 hours postmortem, unless the body was attended to by an inspector or medical professional 24 hours after the person had died.

This legislation also protected medical practitioners who received the corpses. Those who provided the corpse(s) needed to include a certificate including the demographic information of the corpse before it could be turned over to the practitioner. Once they were done with the dissection, the certificate would then be passed on to the inspector. This paperwork was intended to ensure that bodies used for anatomical dissection were no longer exhumed from cemeteries and burial grounds and had been obtained by lawful means. After the medical practitioner had finished dissecting the cadaver, they were responsible for its burial. They were permitted to either wrap the body in a winding cloth, or place it into a coffin prior to burial. It was expected that the body would be "decently interred in consecrated ground, or in some public burial-ground in use for persons of that religious persuasion to which the person whose body was so removed belonged."[69]

The trust broken by the resurrectionists-turned-murderers and the subsequent legal changes had its social effects as well. The Anatomy Act of 1832 was not universally accepted. Doctors, medical professionals, and politicians were concerned that the "Act for Regulating the Schools of Anatomy" would increase the public's mistrust of the medical profession. The editor of the medical journal Lancet, Thomas Wakley, voiced his concerns that the Anatomy Act of 1832 would add to the public's distrust of dissection because the poor would come to believe that their bodies would be sold, rather than donated, and people would profit from their death.[70] As early as 1823 there had been indications that resurrectionists were stealing corpses from the workhouses by pretending to be acquainted with the recently deceased. Upon receipt of the body, the resurrectionists would promptly sell it to an anatomist or school.[71] Much like W. Hunter's request not to be dissected after he died, Sir Astley Cooper's perspectives on the resurrectionists changed over time. Despite the support that he showed regarding the necessity of the resurrectionist's involvement in the study of medicine throughout his lifetime, he was relieved that the need for the profession had waned.

The public's fear of their corpses being sold to anatomists was exemplified when the cholera epidemic struck London in 1832. Medical advancements were still over thirty years from the developments made by Lister and Koch to develop a provable germ theory. Without a provable germ theory, there were misunderstandings about what caused the cholera outbreak. Rumors speculated that the epidemic was planned by the medical community in order to gain more bodies to be dissected. The public theorized that this practice would be enacted by forcing the sick to go "into special hospitals where they could be dissected."[72] The situation was so tense that people began to riot in Manchester when it was discovered that the head of a child, who had died at the Swan Street Cholera Hospital, had been taken and replaced with a brick prior to the burial of the body. The trust that had been built between the public, the medical community, and the resurrectionists had been altered forever. Neither the public, nor the medical community trusted the resurrectionists. Worse, the public no longer trusted the intentions of the medical community. As the importance of the resurrectionists in the medical narrative shifted from recent history to social memory, so too did the acceptance of the trade. Historical scholarship of the middle and late nineteenth century showed a general bias of disgust of the resurrectionist trade. By the early twentieth century, historical scholars wrote about resurrectionism as though it was something that had happened in the long distant past, until the resurrectionist part of the medical narrative drifted into the realms of ghost stories and folklore.

CHAPTER 6

The Medical Community Responds to Misdiagnosed Death

"A servant girl, who had been for some days ill of a fever, to all appearance died, and on Thursday morning was interred in a burying ground in the city. Some hours after she was buried, noise was heard in the grave, which was thereupon immediately dug up, and the body taken out. The girl was alive when the coffin was opened, but expired in a few moments after: Her body was much bruised and scratched from struggling in the grave before she was taken up."[1]

* * *

The first Society for the Recovery of Persons Apparently Dead, was instituted in Amsterdam, Holland. Although the Amsterdam society was only active from 1767 to 1771, the ripples that it caused in Western medicine changed the world. The group focused on ways to use the resuscitative process to help revive people who had stopped breathing, specifically due to suffocation from humidity in the mines, strangulation, choking, stifling, etc.[2] In his pamphlet *A Short Account of a Society at Amsterdam* (1773), Alexander Johnson noted the previous work done on the resuscitative process and advocated for its continued usage in England. He extended the research being done on the resuscitative process by postulating that it could be used to revive people who would were in an apparently dead state, no matter what the cause. He was enthusiastic about the premise that using the resuscitative process during all cases of apparent death would save people who would have otherwise been prematurely buried.

That same year, Johnson proposed that an institution be created in England which focused on "the recovery of persons apparently dead."[3] He relayed the steps that the Society for the Recovery of Persons Apparently

Dead in Amsterdam used for the purpose of resuscitation. He explained that the medical assistant should use "a tobacco pipe, a pair of bellows, or the sheath of a knife" to blow tobacco smoke through the victim's intestines.[4] Once the fumigation of the body was complete, it was considered a best practice to keep the body warm and dry to counter the cold and stiff symptoms of drowning. In addition to using warm blankets and bed-warming pans to keep the body warm, a physician, surgeon, or medical assistant generated friction heat by rubbing their hands over the patient's spine, back, and neck. As the patient exhibited the signs of revival, they were made to sneeze in order to help draw air into the lungs and through the body. Johnson explained that once signs of life were observed, the person could be given strong spirits like wine or brandy, mixed with stimulants like salt, in order to help revive them further. The success of this technique was due to the pungent taste of highly salted liquor, which was intended to shock the system or prompt the victim to expel some of the excess water that may have stagnated in their lungs or stomach. Additionally, Johnson included Tossach's method of resuscitation. Specifically, he indicated the importance of inflating the lungs by "closing off their nose with one hand, and pressing over the left breast with the other," while blowing air into the mouth.[5]

After the dissolution of the Amsterdam Society, several similar societies were instituted throughout Western Europe, including in Italy, Germany, France, and England. In 1774, Drs. William Hawes and Thomas Cogen established the "Institution for Affording Immediate Relief to Persons Apparently Dead from Drowning" in England, which was renamed the Royal Humane Society (RHS) when it received the patronage of King George III in 1787. The 17 founding physicians, and the many who followed, furthered the clinical and practical research of the resuscitative process, provided financial awards to people who attempted to save lives utilizing the resuscitative process and eventually renamed it "cardiopulmonary resuscitation" (CPR). From its inception to 2021, over 88,000 cases have come under the review of the Royal Humane Society committee and over 200,000 awards have been given out.[6] The RHS held annual meetings where members of the Society, members of the general public who had attempted to use the resuscitative process, and those whose lives had been saved through use of the resuscitative process would gather. During the annual meeting of 1793, the Rev. Samuel Glasse delivered a sermon in which he credited the resuscitative process for removing the "morbid affections of the system, [and being] equally active and happy in accomplishing triumphs over the grave."[7] Those involved in the Royal Humane Society of London understood that in order to obtain the maximum effect, it was imperative to teach laymen to accept, learn, and utilize the process.

Their efforts proved to be successful, since over two centuries later the process continues to be taught and utilized throughout the world.

Drowning was a common occurrence in London. The London Bills of Mortality 1700–1758 recorded a range of 45 (1716)–142 (1755) cases, with an average of 84 people dying from drowning annually. According to the RHS, 123 people died due to drowning in 1773. It has been hypothesized that many of the drowning victims either worked on the Thames, which ran through London, or in one of the other lakes or waterways throughout the city. Prior to the acceptance of the resuscitative process there were several other remedies that were commonly used to try to revive those who had appeared to have drowned. At the time, it was believed that people who drowned inhaled or ingested a large amount of water. Therefore, the goal of the earlier remedies was to dispel the water perceived to still be inside of the drowned person. One such remedy placed the body in a supine position over a barrel and rolled the barrel slowly in order to put pressure on the stomach and diaphragm to force the liquid out. Other remedies consisted of suspending the person by wrapping ropes under their arms and legs, or by suspending the person upside down. If the water did not come out easily, the feather of a quill would be thrust down their throat to trigger the gag reflex and cause them to vomit. As more was learned about human physiology and the effects that drowning had on the body, England's medical community began to focus on remedies such as the resuscitative process, which did not have such negative effects on the body.

The 1774 *Proceedings of the Society for the Recovery of the Apparently Drowned* in London presented the steps of the resuscitative process that were expected to be followed by medical professionals. First, it was recommended that the body be handled carefully and that it should not be shaken, hung upside-down, rolled upon the ground, or have the stomach compressed. Rather, "the unfortunate object should be cautiously conveyed by two or more persons or in a carriage upon straw, lying as on a bed with the head a little raised, and kept in as natural and easy a position as possible."[8] In this case, the body was considered to be an "object." Ostensibly this was because the person was believed to be in a state of absolute death, and therefore the soul had become dormant and the consciousness and personality detached from the body. However, the care that was to be taken with the body indicated an awareness that the person may have only entered into an apparently dead state. Therefore, the resuscitative process was attempted until tests for death could be used to determine if the body was in a state of apparent or absolute death. Whether correctly diagnosed as dead, or not, every person who died was considered to have passed through a stage of apparent death. It was not common for the stage of apparent death to be recorded, unless something remarkable happened, such as the person waking back up. Likewise, when a person was diagnosed as dead, the stages of death were not distinctly indicated. Rather it was taken for granted that they had passed through each stage until their ultimate demise.

Once the body was moved to an appropriate location to receive care, those employing the resuscitative process would use a nearby fire, hot water bottles, warming pans, and warm baths to slowly raise the body temperature of the apparently drowned person to just above that of a healthy person. During the eighteenth century, the goal was to raise the body's temperature to a healthy state in order to kickstart their automatic animal functions back into action. After the patient's temperature began to stabilize, one person employing the resuscitative process would close the patients nose with one hand and blow into the patient's mouth. Simultaneously, a second person would start performing chest compressions on the patient's body. Once the lungs had been stimulated, small bellows would be used to administer a tobacco smoke enema and a stimulant would be rubbed on the patient's temples in order to increase the blood flow in the head.

When the person began to rouse, they would be bled immediately to help lower the patient's slightly raised temperature and to keep them calm. Once the patient had been revived and was in a calm state, those applying the resuscitative process would attempt to elicit a sensory response from the patient. The patient's throat and nose would be tickled to make them sneeze or cough. This would ensure that their lungs could both expand and contract. Next, the patient's ability to swallow would be tested by administering increasing increments of liquid, starting with a teaspoon. If the patient remained unresponsive, the medical professional would use small bellows in order to blow air into the bowels or lungs for a short time before declaring the person to be dead.

The creation of the Institution for Affording Immediate Relief to Persons Apparently Dead from Drowning stemmed, in part, from an awareness of the premature burial of people presumed to be dead. Doctors of the time felt that their fears of premature burial were confirmed by the necessity of the resuscitative process and the Institution to study and promote its use. In his *Cautions Against the Burial of Persons Supposed Dead*, RHS co-founder William Hawes explained that it was his "duty" to provide information so that people were not accidentally "being laid out, or, what is more horrible, buried alive."[9] During the mid- to late eighteenth century, the benefits of using the resuscitative process were published in newspapers, in books written by the RHS, and by doctors who believed in its benefits, such as Drs. Alexander Johnson and Anthony Fothergill. In 1789, the

Times published a letter about an additional use of the resuscitative process: to revive an apparently dead person from a state of suffocation rather than asphyxiation. The author of the letter, David Samwell, explained that he had discovered the London printer, James Corrall, unconscious in his shop after suffocating on the smoke of burning coal. By the time Samwell had found him, Corrall had already slipped into a state of apparent death, without any detectable pulse or respiration.[10] Samwell employed the resuscitative process for 15 minutes, after which Corrall began to convulse and revive. As he regained his senses, Samwell gave him some cordial and put him to bed, making sure that his condition was stable before he left. Upon checking up on Corrall the following day, Samwell found that he had made a complete recovery.

Despite the encouraging results of the resuscitative process, it was not readily accepted by all. According to an article published in the *Morning Chronicle*, some people believed that Alexander Johnson's fears regarding the medical community gatekeeping knowledge about the resuscitative process had come to fruition and claimed that only the Humane Society knew how to properly execute the resuscitative process.[11] However, this claim was not rooted in truth. While it was preferable that the medical assistants of the RHS employed the resuscitative process, in instances where no RHS assistants were available, members of the public who were familiar with this revival technique were encouraged to utilize it and were even financially awarded. These rewards were contingent on the use of the resuscitative process, not on whether or not the patient was revived.[12] If the resuscitative process was used unsuccessfully, the RHS awarded the person, who had attempted the technique, two guineas; if its use was successful, the person was awarded four guineas.[13] Johnson published thousands of pamphlets that included practical instructions written for the general public and strongly encouraged widespread application. These pamphlets were disseminated throughout the United Kingdom, throughout the British Empire at large, and even to America.[14] In his *Relief from Accidental Death*, Johnson set the instructions to verse. He explained his intent in providing the instructions in this form as follows:

> The extensive degree of benefit that can arise to the nation from a practice known capable of affording relief in all cases of apparent death, by a treatment sufficiently plain, to be applicable by every person of common ability, is proportionate to the universality of the knowledge of it, and to the number of hands humanely employed in its efficient operations: the number of *medical assistants* proposed by the Humane Societies for this beneficial work, is small, and thinly spread, comparatively to the multitude of men found every where, ready to tender aid on all urgent occasions. The greatest advantage, therefore, that can derive from this practice, must be reaped from the multitude of

hands, not from the confined number to which it is restrained. As the success will likewise depend upon the celerity of applying the means; life, in that suspended state, existing but as a spark.[15]

A snippet of the first stanza in Johnson's verse reads:

> In cases the most common that we meet, (I)
> Ere death the last decisive stroke complete.
> Some time elapses;—yet uncertainty
> Attends that space—it long or short may be:
> Therefore employ that interval to try
> If ye some sparks of life may dormant lie.
> And either a recov'ry safe procure,
> Or from that worst of horrors thus ensure
> Of quick interment. For experience shows,
> That many women, from child-bearing throes,
> And new-born infants, breathless long remain
> Inswooning 'strances,—yet revive again (10.11.12.13)
> By means here recommended.[16]

In the next stanza, he presented familiar ways that should not have been used to revive a person from a variety of issues which would restrict their breathing. Once he had informed the reader of ways that should not be used, he supplied them with information that they could use to rouse an apparently dead person. In the case of drowning, he stated the following:

> At first discov'ry of apparent death,
> Lost not a moment; for the fleeting breath
> May yet be stay'd—while life's last spark remains,
> Patient attend, nor spare or time or pains.
> Avoid the dangerous practice not decry'd,
> By ignorance and prejudice oft try'd,
> Rolling with violence, nor shaking try
> Nor yet suspending—who those means apply
> To force discharge of water, to the grave
> Consign the wretch whom gentler means might save.
> First, from wet cloathes [sic] the body free,—with care
> Wrap it in flannels soft and warm;—beware
> You not sharp salt, nor yet corrosive ply
> Nor rub with wetted cloths, but keep all dry.
> These early steps when taken with the drown'd,
> (On whom success first ascertain'd was found).[17]

Instances where the resuscitative process was utilized by the public were reported in a variety of print sources throughout England after Johnson's book *Relief from Accidental Death; or, Summary Directions, in Verse, Extracted from the Instructions at Large* was published in 1789. Two of them are listed here.

The *Leeds Intelligencer* reported the story of James Roberts, who was found in an apparently dead state near Sheffield. After he was laid out to be buried, he was attended to by "some gentlemen" who used the resuscitative process on him. He revived within three hours and he continued on his way the next morning[18] (December 29, 1789).

The *Chester Chronicle* published the following report of a person who had been prematurely diagnosed as dead:

> A few days since a young man was found apparently dead, near town; some people gathered round the body, and a person was dispatched to the coroner to know what was to be done with the corpse; but before the messenger returned, a worthy clergyman, thinking it not impossible that the common people might be mistaken in what seemed to them the appearance of death, and though a considerable time had elapsed, instantly employed the means of restoration, with success; he was then put into a warm bed, and properly taken care of, and pursued his journey afterwards in health and spirits[19] [April 5, 1793].

This report included a rare follow up, wherein it was stated that

> the long and dangerous suspension of the faculties of the above person, were owing to indigence and fatigue; and, therefore, it is inserted as a caution to the public, not to trust too easily the appearance of death. In a variety of instances the principal vitality is resident in the body, and only requires exertions for the performance of it's [*sic*] wonted and accustomed functions.[20]

In order to achieve the best results, it was expected that the entire resuscitative process would take more than two hours to complete. However, reports of the resuscitative process being practiced between 30–45 minutes were common. These times conflict greatly with the modern understanding of death due to lack of oxygen and the usage of CPR. It is now generally accepted that irreversible brain damage begins after the brain has gone without oxygen for four minutes, with the possibility of death within eight to twelve minutes.[21] Performing resuscitation between four and ten minutes after the disruption of oxygen increases the likelihood that the patient will suffer from memory, coordination, or movement disorders, with the possibility of falling into a "persistent coma" after only a few more minutes.[22] Despite these generalizations, hypothermic conditions can lengthen the survival time to up to 45 minutes after submersion. This occurs because the cold temperature slows down the body's metabolism, which then decreases the amount of oxygen that the body needs to perform its essential functions.

Unfortunately, many of the eighteenth-century reports regarding the use of the resuscitative process and the relative health of the person afterwards do not retain their validity when compared against the modern understanding of anatomy and physiology. It has been generally suggested

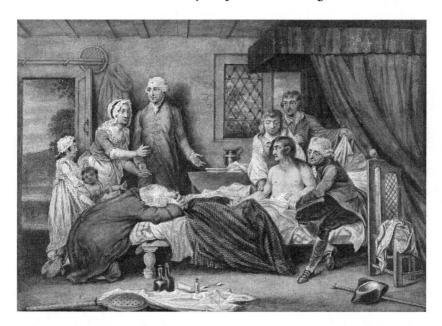

A man recovers due to the use of the resuscitative process after he almost drowned (used with permission from the Wellcome Collection. Attribution 4.0 International [CC BY 4.0]).

that CPR be continued for up to 60 minutes (in children) or until the "victim starts to show signs of regaining consciousness, such as coughing, opening his or her eyes, speaking, or moving purposefully AND starts to breathe normally."[23] A study done in 2015 analyzed the findings of CPR that had been performed on 160 children who had drowned and presented with hypothermia between 1993 and 2012. Of the 98 children who received resuscitation for over 30 minutes, 87 did not survive and the 11 who survived suffered from "severe neurological impairment[s]."[24] Conversely, the children who received resuscitation for under 30 minutes survived with "normal to moderate disability status."[25] The authors explained that the children were more likely to survive the event if it occurred in water temperatures of 0°–46.4°F and they were submersed for less than 30 minutes. Despite the findings of this small study, the authors admitted that they "still have no clear idea about the absolute limits of survival."[26]

During the eighteenth century, doctors did not regularly have or record follow-up appointments with their patients. Likewise, they did not tend to record names in their medical notes, preferring to use the patient's job or closest male relation, for example "the town baker," or "Mr. X's child." Therefore, there are few records from the time that indicate the long-term effects on the patient's health after the use of the resuscitative process. This lack of information includes the long-term effects of procedures such as enemas and bleeding in addition to the respiratory and compression techniques, over the course of 30 minutes to two hours. The few cases that did include follow up reports generally indicated that the process was successful and that the patients continued to live for the vague term of "years" afterwards and were in "perfect health."

Although modern findings differ from those recorded during the eighteenth century, it is important to keep in mind that research relating to the best practices and considerations of the short and long term effects of the resuscitative process were only beginning during the eighteenth century. The findings reported during the eighteenth century represented the beginning of empirical study; therefore, it should be expected that both the studies and their results would differ from studies done in the twenty-first century. These differences are due to the advancement of both medical theory and medical technology. Analysis and theories during the eighteenth and early nineteenth centuries were being created while medical professionals were still in the early and intermediate stages of understanding different parts of human anatomy and physiology. Therefore, these modern statistics and understanding have been presented as a point of contrast, not as an attempt to downplay or negate the progress made during the eighteenth century.

* * *

Even as the medical community worked to save lives by adopting and teaching the resuscitative process, they were still aware that people were being buried alive. During the late eighteenth and early nineteenth centuries, several educated men around Europe speculated about the number of people who had accidentally been buried alive due to being misdiagnosed as dead. In his 1793 sermon in favor of the Royal Humane Society, Dr. Samuel Glasse presented two hypotheses which set the range of people who had been prematurely buried between 10 percent and 50 percent of all deaths. Both of his hypotheses came from French sources: Baron de Hupch (naturalist) and Francois Thieurey (Doctor Regent of the Faculty of Paris, France). De Hupch hypothesized that "of one hundred persons apparently dead, and precipitately interred, ten of them at least may be restored to life, their friends, and their country."[27] Thieurey's hypothesis was considerably higher, putting the number of people who were misdiagnosed as dead and prematurely buried at one-third to one-half of all reported deaths.[28] During the following century, the British mathematician, John Snart surmised that one person out of every ten (10 percent) were being prematurely buried in England, and he wrote an impassioned plea to Parliament on the subject.[29] In 2001, Dr. Jan Bondeson surmised that the statistics reported on the prevalence of premature burial in Western Europe throughout the nineteenth and early twentieth centuries were "highly exaggerated."[30] Bodenson believed that if the literature relating to apparent death and premature burial was reviewed thoroughly, the results would support the views of those who were skeptical about its prevalence during the nineteenth century.[31] The general consensus of skeptics during and after the late nineteenth century was that the percentage of people who were prematurely buried spanned from less than 1 percent to 10 percent. However, until this study, a collection of narratives and stories relating to the misdiagnosis of death and the following consequences has been absent from the scholarship.

Laws and traditions regulating the exhumation of bodies have not typically allowed for a large-scale cemetery exhumation, which has curbed the ability to discover incidences of premature burial across England during the eighteenth century. The Museum of London Archeology (MOLA) has undertaken the exhumation, preservation, and/or relocation of several cemeteries in and around London. These cemeteries date from as far back as the pre–Roman era and as late as the nineteenth century. Their findings are kept within the Osteological Database, which is housed by the Centre for Human Bioarcheology and the Museum of London. The database includes historical context that both describes and provides photographs of the general position and state of the bodies when they were buried. It also includes descriptions of the cemeteries and excavation sites where the bodies were found. Despite the comprehensive data contained within the Osteological Database, it does not include information regarding the placement of the bones. There is no indication if any skeletons were found arranged in an atypical position from burial practices of the time. This is likely because as the body decomposes, it liquifies and disintegrates, "leaving skeletonized remains articulated by ligaments."[32] This means that even if a person had struggled within their coffin during the eighteenth century, unless that coffin was airtight, a modern exhumation would reveal disjointed bones rather than a twisted figure. Because of this, evidence of misdiagnosed death and any subsequent premature repercussions—for the time being—has to be taken from textual and literary evidence such as books and newspapers from the eighteenth century, nineteenth, and twentieth centuries.

By surveying medical texts, the annual reports of the Royal Humane Society, pamphlets, and newspaper articles that were published in Britain, I have identified 200 cases of misdiagnosed death that were reported as occurring between 1700 and 1800. The identified cases were included in books written on premature burial, the resuscitative process, and the understanding of death. Additionally, the selected medical texts either emphasized that death was not well understood or that anatomical understanding was being improved upon to keep people from being prematurely buried in the future. During the eighteenth century, people received most of their local news through newspapers, and many newspapers published stories relating to the misdiagnosis of death and the different premature repercussions that followed. Likewise, pamphlets such as *The Surprising Wonder of Doctor Watts, who lay in a trance three days* (1710), *A new prophesy: Or, An Account of a young Girl, not above Eight Years of Age Who being in a trance, or lay as dead for the Space of 48 Hours* (1780), or those distributed by the RHS and Alexander Johnson were handed out to warn the community that people were being prematurely buried, or to explain to people what to do if someone happened upon a person who was apparently dead. (A list of the books, pamphlets, and the newspapers used are listed in the appendix.)

The people represented in these cases were not necessarily diagnosed by medical professionals but were considered to be in a state of suspended animation, apparent death, or dead by those who first attended to them. Repercussions suffered due to these misdiagnoses included being prematurely enclosed in a coffin, buried in their grave, interred in a tomb, and in some cases dissected after the resurrectionists had delivered their corpse to the medical community. Premature enclosure referred to the person being enclosed in their coffin or winding sheet. By extension, it also included the time that the body spent in the coffin at the wake or at the funeral. Premature burial or interment indicated the next step in the burial process. In these cases, the body would have been moved into the grave, tomb, vault, or mausoleum. Premature dissection occurred when the body was brought to the medical community to be dissected and awoke during the process. It can be assumed that for a body to have been prematurely dissected it had already been misdiagnosed as dead, plus at least one of the other three repercussions. However, the preceding repercussion was not consistently recorded. That is to say, it is not necessarily known if the person who was sold to the medical community was exhumed, disinterred, or stolen during the watching period. Similar to how the Université de la Méditerranée's report that pins were stuck into the toes of the apparently dead indicates that pin implementation was used as a test for death, the casual reference to the resuscitative process in news articles indicates that the theory of resuscitation was accepted by both the medical community and the public at large. Unfortunately, only a few cases included any kind of follow up information. Most reports were single-situational, reflecting what was observed, witnessed or heard about during one interaction with the person.

When it was discovered that a person had been incorrectly diagnosed as dead and suffered a premature repercussion, there were four outcomes:

revival, exhumation, resurrection, or resuscitation. The person was considered to have revived if they transitioned back to life on their own prior to being buried. Many instances of revival occurred before or during the time that the person was enclosed in their coffin. In cases where the person died within their grave or tomb, it was labeled as an exhumation because the body was exhumed—at least temporarily—in order to verify that death had initially been misdiagnosed. Bodies that were brought out of the grave, tomb, or mausoleum alive were labeled as being resurrected. However, after a person was resurrected, their survival was not ensured. In some cases, the person had become too weak to survive by the time help arrived, or the help that was provided was not enough to restore them to health. Cases where the person had revived after they received the resuscitative process were labeled as having been resuscitated. Like those who were resurrected, although the person was roused after being resuscitated, their survival was not guaranteed. Whether or not the person survived is indicated in the section which summarizes each case.

Like the hypotheses reported by Glasse and Snart, the cases surveyed did not necessarily occur in Britain. They were, however, published in British sources and presented to the British public. Cases of people who had been declared as apparently dead and what premature repercussions followed, if any, were analyzed. The following information was collected from each case, as applicable. Demographic information consisted of their name, gender, age range, socio-economic class, and location that the case took place. The race of these cases is assumed to be white because no other race was identified in the sources. Although not all of the demographic and burial information could be collected from each case, all of the cases were analyzed in order to provide the most relevant preliminary information for this study. Areas with missing or incomplete information were regarded cautiously. If a case did not indicate a certain repercussion or revival, it was assumed that none had occurred. If the exact year was not given, but the case indicated that it happened a variable number of years prior to the publication of the written record, that number of years was subtracted from the book's publication date. Similarly, if a description that identified the number of years between the case and the source's publication date was not given, the year of the source's publication was used. Books that were written for the sole purpose of showing the positive effects of the resuscitative process, such as those published by the Royal Humane Society, were reviewed, and their bias was considered before cases were included. If the reported case did not include identifying information on the person, location, or the situation that occurred, it was not included.

When the cases were reviewed per decade, it was noticed that the number of cases reported steadily increased over the course of the eighteenth century. Three were reported during the early decades (1700–1710 and 1711–1720) and the most cases (83) were reported between 1791 and 1800. The only outlier decade was 1751–1760, for which only three reported cases were identified.

The base findings indicated that of the 200 cases of misdiagnosed death, 132 were male, 61 were female, and seven were unspecified. These findings have been delineated by age range, specifically "adult," "child," and "infant." Despite the understanding that children as young as eight were permitted to work during the eighteenth century, the parameters for these designations are based on modern standards: 0 months to 1 year old is an infant, 1 year to 17 years of age is a child, and 18-plus years of age is an adult. According to these findings, the majority of people who were misdiagnosed as dead were adult males.

	Infant	Child	Adult	Unspecified
Male	3	33	93	3
Female	0	15	45	1
Unspecified	2	4	1	0
Total	5	52	139	4

Table 1: Age Ranges of the Misdiagnosed Dead (200 Cases)

The cases of apparent death routinely included a location. While some cases were specific enough to include a town or waterway, all except nine of them indicated the country where the incident occurred. Despite the cases being published in British sources, they did not all occur in England or the United Kingdom. The recorded cases occurred throughout Europe, in British military outposts, and in America. The American and military-based cases were included due to their extended connections to England. It is plausible that the increased prevalence of reported cases occurred in England, either because the author was British or to make the subject more relatable to a British audience. Here is the list of countries from which cases were reported in British sources and the number of cases located from each country.

- England (125) and its military ships/outposts (5)
- France (18)
- Ireland (11)
- Scotland (11)
- Germany/Prussia (10)
- America (3)
- Holland/Netherlands (2)
- Italy (2)
- Spain (2)
- Austria (1)
- Hungary (1)
- Sweden (1)
- Wales (1)
- Unspecified (7)

The results of this study were analyzed both inclusively and by show-casing the numbers specifically from England. The inclusive results revealed that of the 200 cases, 29 or 14.5 percent of the people who were misdiagnosed as dead suffered a premature repercussion; of that 14.5 percent, 55 percent of them had been prematurely buried or interred. Of the total 29 people were incorrectly diagnosed as dead, and the following premature repercussions were experienced: buried in their grave (14), enclosed in their coffin (11), interred in their tomb (two), or dissected (two). The survival rates of those who experienced a premature repercussion were also evaluated. Those who were prematurely enclosed in their coffin had the best rate of survival at nearly 90 percent; only one person died. Half of the people who were prematurely buried or prematurely interred survived. Finally, half of the people who were prematurely dissected survived. Of the 29 people who were misdiagnosed as dead and incurred a premature repercussion as a result, a majority (65.5 percent) survived the encounter.

Outcome	Enclosed (11)	Buried (14)	Interred (2)	Dissected (2)
Survived	10	7	1	1
Died	1	7	1	1

**Table 2: Premature Repercussions by Type
and Survival Rate in Inclusive Cases (200)**

One hundred and thirty (65 percent) of the collected cases of mis-diagnosed death were reported as having occurred in England or on a British ship/outpost. In these cases, 89 were reported as males, 37 were females, and four were of an unspecified gender.

	Infant	Child	Adult	Unspecified
Male	2	26	61	0
Female	0	8	28	1
Unspecified	0	4	0	0
Total	2	38	89	1

Table 3: Age Ranges of the Misdiagnosed Dead in England (130 Cases)

Of these 130 cases, seven people suffered a premature repercussion. Four people were prematurely enclosed in their coffin, three were prematurely buried, none were prematurely interred, and none were prematurely dissected. All of the people who were prematurely enclosed in their coffin survived, and two of the people who were prematurely buried died. Due to the low rate of premature repercussions that befell those who were

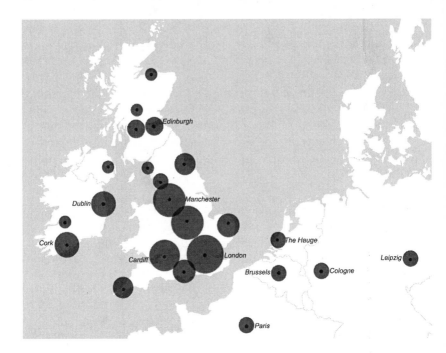

Cases of misdiagnosed death reported in England within 25 miles of major cities (map created by Erika Morton).

incorrectly diagnosed as dead in England, the survival rate was nearly 99 percent.

Outcome	Enclosed (4)	Buried (3)	Interred (0)	Dissected (0)
Survived	4	1	—	—
Died	0	2	—	—

**Table 4: Premature Repercussions by Type
and Survival Rate of Cases in England (130)**

When this data on cases of misdiagnosed death is compared against the hypotheses on the amount of people who were prematurely buried, as supplied by Glasse (10 percent to 50 percent in Western Europe) and Snart (10 percent in England), it is important to keep in mind that 200 cases is a relatively small sample size. Unfortunately, neither Glasse, de Hupch, Thieurey, or Snart reported the number of people included in their hypotheses. Therefore, if all of the hypotheses are considered to be equal, the findings from this study suggested that the total amount of people who suffered a premature repercussion (14.5 percent) favor de Hupch and Snart's hypotheses that 10 percent of people were being prematurely buried. This is especially noticeable when the 55 percent of people who were prematurely buried or interred is applied to the 14.5 percent of the total (200 people) who experienced a premature repercussion; 55 percent of 14.5 percent equals just under 8 percent. It also emphasizes how exaggerated Thieurey's approximation that 33.3 percent to 50 percent of people who were diagnosed as dead were being prematurely buried appears, especially since his theories only related to the prevalence of premature burial/interment. This validates some of the moderate estimates regarding the percentage of people being prematurely buried across Europe during the eighteenth century. The difference between the results of this study and the theory of Thieurey also validates Dr. Bondeson's supposition that guestimates from the era were high. Since a more robust sample size would require an archeological project, these statistics from my study are only preliminary. Continued research regarding the misdiagnosis of death and subsequent repercussions throughout eighteenth-century Europe will be necessary to produce a more comprehensive analysis.

CHAPTER 7

Nineteenth Century
Scholars Weigh In

A cook's apprentice in Paris, France, appeared to be dead, and those close to him began to prepare him for burial. As the coffin began to be lowered into his grave, a noise could be heard coming from inside of it. The lid was quickly opened, and the apprentice sat up as though he had just awoken from a nightmare. "My God! Do I still dream?" he asked.[1] *Although he was alive when he was removed from the coffin, the situation gave him quite a shock, and those closest to him were uncertain if he would completely recover.*

* * *

While the medical community researched the transition from life to death and worked to properly define it, the public's awareness of premature repercussions due to misdiagnosed death increased. British newspapers published hundreds of articles which mentioned that people were "apparently dead" or "had the appearance of death" and the consequences of those appearances. From waking during the watching period to being exhumed alive or twisted-up from struggling inside their coffin or tomb, the British public were able to read about premature burials as they occurred throughout Europe and America. An article published in the *Ipswich Journal* in 1749 reported on concerns of people dying suddenly in Rome, Italy, and the apprehensions that "some of those people might be buried alive."[2]

In addition, the British press legitimized these fears by publishing articles regarding the lengths that people went to in order to prevent being buried alive. An article in the *Newcastle Chronicle* in July 1768, took a macabre turn when a woman bequeathed £50 to her surgeon "on the condition that he cuts her throat as soon as she has been dead twelve hours."[3] The author of this article left no question as to why the woman made that request by including the statement that "the fear of being buried alive has occasioned this legacy."[4] A similar story was reported in the June 6, 1791, edition of the *Derby Mercury* wherein it stated that Lady Dryden pre-paid a surgeon "to cut her throat, before the interment of her corpse; which operation, we understand, has been duly performed agreeably to her ladyship's desire."[5] Reports like these indicated that people were aware that mistakes were being made regarding properly diagnosing death and their fears related to premature burial. The fear of what would happen to them after they transitioned to an apparently dead state appeared to scare them more than the actual act of dying. The following excerpt from a letter published in the *Northampton Mercury* in September 1791 explained the fears associated with waking up buried in one's grave:

> Too many have been buried alive whole Dissolution appeared sudden, and who were not kept a proper Time: Conceive the accumulated Horrors of such a Condition; a Man awakes in the Prison of the Grave, perhaps in his full Strength; he is cut off for ever from every tender Connection which attached him to Life, oppressed with his most horrid Situation, stung with the keenest Hunger, and apprehensive of an approaching Eternity.[6]

As it became known that people were being misdiagnosed as dead and then were being closed within their coffin—if not worse—two public responses began to emerge. The first was an acceptance that this problem was occurring followed by an interest in finding a solution. The second was a dismissal of the growing concerns of receiving a premature diagnosis of death and the subsequent repercussions, claiming that they were alarmist in nature.

The concept of apparent death also took on two meanings during the eighteenth century. In some cases the British press printed articles relating to violent assaults, murders, and mining accidents and utilized the term "apparently dead" to describe the state of the victims and provided no further information regarding their recovery. In other cases "apparent death" or "apparently dead" was the actual witness-driven diagnosis which was then followed by an attempt to revive the person or indicated that burial preparations would begin. The casual usage of the terms "apparently dead" and "apparent death" indicated that British society had accepted it as a transitional stage that occurred when someone no longer appeared to be living. In the following news article, published in the June 23, 1798, edition of the *Hampshire Chronicle*, an unnamed woman appeared to have died, and the body was put aside until it was time for it to be buried. When a doctor looked at the body, he noticed that she was still showing signs of life and called off the burial, which had been scheduled for the following day. About a week later, the woman revived.

> Singular Case. About a fortnight since, a woman aged about 60, in the workhouse belonging to Greenwich, was suddenly struck with apparent death and

was ordered to be buried on the Sunday following; accordingly, she was put into her coffin, and taken into the place where the dead are kept till buried; but on Saturday morning, the Doctor of the workhouse going to look at her, saw symptoms that induced him to forbid her burial that day. He visited her every day after till Friday, leaving the same order; but, to the astonishment of every person, on Friday, about the same time she had been taken on that day week, she suddenly rose up in her coffin, and is still alive.[7]

By calling off the burial, the doctor had stopped the woman from suffering the premature repercussions of being prematurely enclosed in her coffin and then buried. Waiting to enclose an apparent corpse into a coffin was crucial because there was a finite amount of time—approximately six hours—in which a person could be rescued after the top was affixed shut. After that, the person inside would asphyxiate. One of the most poignant signs that the British public took concerns about a living person being prematurely enclosed in their coffin seriously was the creation of the safety coffin.

Safety coffins were coffins that included a way for those enclosed within to signal to people on the outside of the coffin that they were still alive. Descriptions of people being twisted up in their winding sheets, their hands and feet bloodied from kicking against the ends of the coffin or pounding on the lid, their extremities and torsos torn into as they panicked, were published in books, pamphlets, and news articles throughout the eighteenth and nineteenth centuries. These reports increased the public's awareness and fears. One of the most famous accounts of a safety coffin was that of the Duke of Brunswick. Prior to his death in 1792, the Duke was so worried about being buried alive that he ordered the creation of an elaborate safety coffin. More than just a way to indicate that he was alive, his coffin included means to keep him alive until he could be rescued. This included a way to deliver food and a pipe to deliver fresh air. Unfortunately, the science of the time had not advanced to the point of understanding the theories of air and oxygen flow. Even if the Duke had been enclosed in his coffin and buried alive, he would have still run out of breathable air in approximately six hours because the tube designed to keep the air fresh would have filled with his own carbon dioxide, as he exhaled.

The safety coffin is often ascribed to being a late eighteenth-century/ early nineteenth-century invention. However, an article published in the *Derby Mercury*, on May 3, 1733, reported that the Suffolk lawyer, John Frohock "always had a terrible Apprehension of being buried alive."[8] In order to assuage his fears, he requested that a special coffin be made with the following specifications:

the Lid of the Coffin in which he is to be put, shall be made with Hinges to open easily; and that four Persons be appointed continually to attend his corpse, not only before 'tis buried, but for Eight Days after Interment in his

Vault; in which Time if he should happen to come to Life, he intends to rap against the Coffin-Lid, and his Attendants are in such case to furnish their proper Assistance.[9]

Frohock's request to have hinges on his coffin predated the Duke by about sixty years. Since his reason for putting hinges on his coffin lid was to allow for the ease of his release, he had, effectively, furnished the precursor to the safety coffin.

By the end of the eighteenth century, the concept of the safety coffin had spread to other countries in Europe. In 1798, the German priest P.G. Pessler suggested that all coffins buried in a churchyard should have a way to notify the living that someone had returned to consciousness after being buried. He indicated that each coffin should have a hollow tube connected to it with a rope encased, which connected the apparently dead person to the church bells.[10] He theorized that as the person who had been prematurely buried moved within their coffin, they would shake the cord and ring the church bells, thus alerting people that they were still alive. Unfortunately, the idea was better in theory than in reality. In reality, the plan would fall apart due to mechanical incongruities. The cord that would need to be used would have to be small enough to fit inside the coffin and be easily shaken with enough force that the vibration would travel a considerable distance and still forceful enough to ring the church bell.

Safety coffins continued to be developed during the nineteenth century. When the topic of safety coffins is discussed, people tend to envision a small-scale version of Pessler's idea, with a string emerging from the grave, attached to a bell supported by a shepherd's crook. However, that construction is unrealistic because the weight of the compacted dirt would not allow a string to gain enough motion to ring a bell. The safety coffin patent that looks the most similar to the description was granted to Dr. Johann Taberger in 1829. Taberger's safety coffin had a metal cord that was attached to the corpse's wrist or ankle and was encased in a tube that connected to a bell on the other end.

The Central Cemetery Museum in Vienna, Austria, has a safety coffin bell rig from the nineteenth century. Rather than a string, there is a metal cord that would attach to the foot of the corpse and then to a hammered bell, resembling a fire bell, which was encased in a wooden box. If someone had been buried while they were in an apparently dead state and regained consciousness in the grave, they could kick their feet, causing the cord to shake and the bell to clang. The clanging would then alert the cemetery watchmen that someone had been buried alive. Unfortunately, this design had a fatal flaw: the body naturally moves as it decomposes. Therefore, it has been widely accepted that there were instances where the decomposing

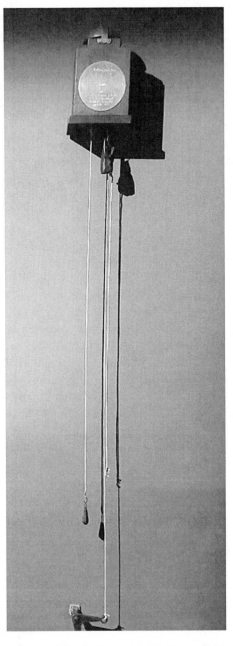

Safety coffin from the Central Cemetery Museum in Vienna, Austria (used with permission from the Central Cemetery Museum; photograph by the author).

dead were exhumed due to false alarms sounding out across cemeteries.

Although safety coffins with the bell attached is arguably the most well-known design, other options were available. During the late eighteenth century, the doctor Rev. Robert Robinson was so afraid of being prematurely buried that he requested "a glass window to be placed in his coffin over his face, in order that any signs of life exhibited after burial might be detected."[11] For many years after his death in 1791 crowds would visit his grave, first to see if he decomposed and, later, to see that he had. After some time had passed, "morbid curiosity" of these visitors became bothersome and his grave was filled.[12] While sliding glass panels into the coffin lid were not commonplace during the eighteenth century, this idea gained in popularity during the nineteenth century. As early as the 1820s, coffins began to be made out of metal with glass panels put into the lid. This allowed the living to watch the dead for decomposition. If the enclosed body did not decompose, these panels allowed people to watch for any signs of life without reopening the coffin. Metal coffins also had the benefit of being able to house ice in a compartment below the chamber that held the body. This allowed for slightly longer preservation of the body, especially during the warmer months.

One safety coffin of note was the Eisenbrandt Life Preserving Coffin, which the patent states was "to be used in cases of doubtful death."[13] This coffin was patented in 1843 and allowed a person who was prematurely enclosed into their coffin to free themselves without assistance. The only caveat was that the person needed to awaken prior to burial. This coffin had a small springboard inside that would be compressed when the body's shoulders lay on top. It also had a thin rod of metal that was screwed horizontally to the interior of the coffin and was positioned over the torso of the body. The rod was connected to a latch with a thin piece of curved metal affixed to the inside top rim of the coffin. If the rod opened the latch, that thin piece of metal would allow for the lid to pop up or swing open. As the body moved forward, the springboard would decompress, pushing the body out of the coffin. The company described their corpse ejection system as superior to other safety coffins that were on the market. An advertisement for the Eisenbrandt Life Preserving Coffin read that "the *slightest* motion of its inmate will be instantly communicated to the springs, which freeing the coffin-lid, it flies open—a circumstance which entirely relieves the confinements of the body, and thus removes all uneasiness of premature interment from the minds of anxious friends and relatives."[14] The premise behind the Life Preserving Coffin was a good one. However, if the body moved because the coffin had been jostled or because it started to decompose, the sensitivity of the design could have resulted in bodies randomly popping out of coffins.

* * *

While the availability of various forms of safety coffins signaled the public's genuine concern about being buried alive, there was a subsection of people who believed that these fears were overstated. In his often contradictory dissertation, *Disorder of Death*, Walter Whiter explained that unnamed "alarmists" were interested in "delaying Interment, till Putrefaction the supposed sign of absolute Death appears."[15] Whiter used the word "alarmist" to reference people who were *overly* concerned about cases of misdiagnosed death resulting in premature burial. He admitted that people were genuinely concerned about the prospect about being buried alive and that there was a possibility that it could happen. However, he thought that people who focused on warning others of the dangers of premature burial should have, instead, focused their efforts on adding to the scholarship on why and how people were being misdiagnosed as dead to begin with. He believed that those who focused specifically on preventing premature burial played on the public's fears about the phenomenon and caused undue panic. Additionally, he theorized that the number of people who were prematurely buried was so low that there was no need to wait until the body had showed signs of putrefaction before burying it. Instead, he surmised that those who waited until the body had begun to rot did so to assuage their own concerns about ensuring that the person was dead and would not revive. He considered their focus on the death, rather than the revival of the individual, to be "perverted conceptions."[16] In this way, his perspective was limited, because he viewed each situation of a person reviving from an apparently dead state as an independent case rather than an indication that several instances could create a concerning trend.

Towards the end of the nineteenth century there was a resurgence of societal and academic interests relating to the handling of the corpse. Society's relationship with death had evolved alongside the advancement of medical theory throughout the nineteenth century. During the 1890s, the focus shifted beyond solidifying the definition of death to include the treatment of the corpse. In 1893, the Select Committee submitted recommendations to the House of Commons to regulate the certification of death. They recommended that the cause of death be observed and recorded on each death certificate and that this certificate could only be produced by "registered medical practitioner[s], or by a coroner after inquest, or, in Scotland, by a procurator fiscal."[17] If a medical practitioner could not see the body themselves, then two people who personally knew the deceased could sign the certificate verifying that the person had died. Additionally, the Select Committee recommended that "a registered medical practitioner should be appointed as public medical certifier of the cause of death in cases in which a certificate from a medical practitioner in attendance was not forthcoming."[18] After the death certificate had been completed, it was to be given to the death registrar instead of being given to the deceased's family. The registrar would then inform the family of where and how the body could be properly buried. After the family had received this information, they would need to dispose of the body within a period of eight days from the time of death. If they held onto the body longer than the eight day period, then they could be charged with a penal offense. This process was not perfect and approximately 11,464 unverified deceased bodies were buried in England in 1905.[19] However, these changes regulated the process of verifying death and allowed for the formalized legislation that followed during the twentieth century.

The evolution of medical theory during the nineteenth century resulted in debates about the validity of studying premature burial as an academic pursuit. The doctors William Tebb and Colonel Edward Vollum believed that premature burial continued to be a valid concern and sought to educate the public about the issue with their book *Premature Burial and*

How It May Be Prevented. The book provided a historical perspective on the issue and included stories, mostly pulled from newspapers and journals, regarding people who had been—or had nearly been—prematurely buried throughout Europe due to the improper diagnosis of death. The first edition was published in 1896 and drew both supporters and critics. One vocal critic was Dr. David Walsh, who believed that Tebb and Vollum's fears were alarmist in nature. Walsh based his opinion on the medical understanding of the day. However, he failed to consider any personal experiences relating to the misdiagnosis of death and premature burial, as well as the enormous differences in medical theory and technology between the beginning and end of the nineteenth century.

William Tebb was a social reformer who had spent his life protecting vulnerable and underserved populations. Over the course of his lifetime, he advocated for the abolition of slavery, women's rights, and the kinder treatment of animals. Towards the end of his career, he turned his focus toward what he considered to be the most vulnerable population: the dead. Considering the corpse the victim, he worked to raise awareness regarding diseases and sleep disorders that masqueraded as death. Mirroring the theories of Charles Kite, Tebb theorized that the difference between apparent death and real death was the existence of the "presence of a force or power continually opposed to the action of physical and chemical laws."[20] In other words, the soul. He explained that the presence of such a force indicated that the person was in a state of apparent death and the absence of it indicated that the person's death was absolute. Tebb confirmed that the primary signs of death that had been identified during the eighteenth century were still viable. He explained that an absence of heartbeat, respiration, blood circulation, and nervous response were the general signs of death. He also wrote about the occurrence of rigor mortis but warned that it was not a reliable sign of death. Like the physicians of the eighteenth century, he believed that the only true indication that a person was absolutely dead was putrefaction. He also continued to develop the definition of death to include signs of false death, which he also called death counterfeit. He defined false death/death counterfeit as an advanced state of apparent death which was so profound that the body did not respond to the tests for life.

William Tebb's friend and co-author Colonel Edward Vollum was a doctor who worked as a medical inspector for the United States Army and had served in the Army of the Potomac during the Civil War. Vollum had, personally, been diagnosed as dead after an extended bout of suspended animation due to drowning. He regained consciousness as his body was being prepared for interment. This experience piqued Vollum's curiosity about how people could be mistakenly diagnosed as dead. In response, he wrote prolifically to both the American and British press where "he strongly deprecated the custom of hastily judging by appearances, maintaining that putrefactive decomposition was the only sure proof of death."[21] The public and academic awareness of this issue in the nineteenth century reached a crossroads in 1896 when William Tebb and Edward Vollum instituted the London Association for the Prevention of Premature Burial, the purpose of which was to devise better ways to prevent premature burial and to disseminate information regarding why it happened and how to prevent future cases.

As medical theory and technology advanced, the medical community's response to the continued reports of premature burial continued to advance as well. Rather than considering premature burial to be a frightfully common occurrence, other physicians doubted the validity of the topic as an academic pursuit. Tebb's critic Dr. David Walsh did not consider premature burial a worth academic pursuit. Walsh's medical interests focused on issues that were considered to be diseases of the skin, such as wounds, male baldness, sexually transmitted diseases, and the deep tissue damage that occurred from the use of x-rays. His research was well-respected, and he was appointed as a physician at the Western Skin Hospital of London. He wrote his own book, *Premature Burial: Fact or Fiction* (1897), as a counter-response to Tebb's decidedly historical and informational perspective on premature burial in Western Europe. Walsh's book included medical and academic facts that were known by the end of the nineteenth century. His stance on the significance of the study of misdiagnosed death and its relation to premature burial was predicated on the following idea:

> it may be at once stated that the whole theory of premature burial is unsupported by a single scientifically proved instance; that the likelihood of such an occurrence is extremely small; that the balance of probabilities weighs all in the other direction; in short that the whole of this popular belief is nothing more than a legend.[22]

Despite Walsh's knowledge of Victorian medicine, he neglected to consider how much British society and medicine had evolved between the time of Whiter (1819), the inception of the Anatomy Act of 1832, and the late Victorian era, when these debates of the validity of premature burial as an academic pursuit were taking place. The medical standards that Walsh was accustomed to were vastly advanced from those of the eighteenth and early nineteenth centuries. Tobacco fell out of favor as a trusted medicine at the beginning of the century. The acceptance of the germ theory, in the 1860s, had given the medical community a new understanding of disease transmission and infection. Improved sanitation in London caused people to live longer, and the growth of industry allowed people to improve their quality of life. Scientific and medical theories and understanding developed in the areas of histology, microbiology, pathology, the neuromuscular system, anesthesia, and surgical sterilization, as well as other areas of anatomy and physiology.

Walsh exemplified his ignorance of social and medical history relating to the misdiagnosis of death in *Premature Burial: Fact or Fiction* when he discussed the probability of confusing a sleep disorder with death. It was his opinion that the "trained and careful observer" would notice that the body was still warm and the person was still breathing.[23] He went on to explain that medical attendants verified death in England and if an attendant could not be secured then an inquiry would be held by the coroner. The simplicity of his statements indicated that Walsh did not consider who was verifying death, what training they had to do so, and what theories they were basing their assumptions on during the preceding centuries.

He also took the watching period for granted when he wrote, "Here in England, the body of a dead person is kept five days to a week," during which time he expected that a person would show signs of death.[24] Walsh made no indication that he understood the history or purpose of waiting that length of time. Whiter had discussed this in 1819, explaining that any delay in the burial process tended to be either at the behest of the family or accidental in nature. Walsh analyzed several stories of those who awoke from an apparently dead state and considered them to be either unreliable or alarmist. He was also skeptical of any stories in which the person awoke after being enclosed in their coffin, because by the late nineteenth-century coffins were "air-tight" and anyone who had been prematurely enclosed in their coffin would have suffocated after 10–15 minutes.[25] He did not consider that historically and through the nineteenth-century coffins had largely been made of wood, by hand, and not of the soundness and quality that he was accustomed to seeing. Nor, did he consider that, historically, only those of particular wealth could afford to be buried in a coffin; people of other economic classes were buried in only their winding sheet or shroud. George K. Behlmer's holistic approach on that topic in his article "Grave Doubts: Victorian Medicine, Moral Panic, and the Signs of Death" added that there had not been any authenticated cases of premature burial "unearthed in a generation."[26] The indication that proven cases of premature burial had not been reported in so long means that they had fallen out of social memory, which may have added to Walsh's skepticism. This would also explain why Walsh was not alone in his skepticism of the topic. In fact, Tebb, himself, stated that "the great majority of the medical profession in this country [England] are either skeptical or apathetic as to the alleged danger of living burial."[27]

Walsh made the same mistake of applying late Victorian medical theory to pre–Victorian circumstances by describing the signs of death as they had been recorded by the doctor Sir Benjamin Ward Richardson (1828–1896). Richardson was a Fellow of the Royal Society and the Royal College of Physicians. He had been awarded the Fothergill gold medal by the Medical Society of London (1854) and the Astley Cooper prize awarded by Guy's Hospital (1856). Richardson was well-known for his work in anesthetics, especially chloroform, and was able to identify signs of death that expanded on the cessation of brain, heart, and lung functions. Since it was still difficult to confirm absolute death, the absence of at least two of these symptoms needed to be observed before a person could be considered as apparently dead.

Richardson was considered to be the authority on defining death in late nineteenth-century England. He published a list of eleven signs of death in his *The Absolute Signs and Proofs of Death* (1889). Walsh considered Richardson to be a "logical man" and included the following summarization of Richardson's signs of death in his book:

1. Respiratory failure, including absence of arterial pulsation, of cardiac motion, and of cardiac sounds.
2. Cardiac failure, including absence of arterial pulsation, of cardiac motion, and of cardiac sounds.
3. Absence of turgescence of filling of the veins on making pressure between them and the heart.
4. Reduction of the temperature of the body below the national standard.
5. Rigor mortis and muscular collapse.
6. Coagulation of the blood.
7. Putrefactive decomposition.
8. Absence of red colour in semi-transparent parts under the influence of a powerful stream of light.
9. Absence of muscular contraction under the stimulus of galvanism, of heat, and of puncture.
10. Absence of red blush of the skin after subcutaneous injection of ammonia (Monteverdi's test).
11. Absence of signs of rush or oxidation of a bright steel blade, after plunging it deep into the tissues (the needle test of Cloque and Laborde).[28]

It is evident in observing the differences between the signs and symptoms of death as recorded by Richardson and those developed during the eighteenth century that Walsh took for granted the availability of his accustomed technologies and medical understanding. The "national standard" body temperature, that was indicated in #4, referred to the common physiological understanding about body temperature was developed during the 1860s when Carl Wunderlich analyzed the body temperature of 25,000 people and observed that the average body temperature was 37°C (98.6°F).[29] Richardson theorized that the body temperature of a dead person would be the same inside the mouth as the temperature of the air around the body. Since this standard, as well as the techniques to detect several of Richardson's signs of death (cardiac motion, cardiac sounds, coagulation of blood, injections of ammonia, etc.) had not been developed prior to the nineteenth century, it was unrealistic of Walsh to assume that those who declared the death of others in the preceding centuries would have the same observational awareness and medical knowledge as he was afforded due to his Victorian-era education and scholarship.

In 1899, James R. Williamson wrote a letter to the editor of *The Metaphysical Magazine for the Library* which supported Tebb's concerns and the necessity of the London Association for the Prevention of Premature Burial. While the letter mentioned David Walsh's criticisms of Tebb's stance, it also explained that premature burials continued to occur because the attending doctors were not obligated to verify the disease or provide a death certificate of the person who had apparently died.[30] It went on to explain that a law would be going before Parliament, with the intent of directing physicians to verify that a person showed signs of death prior to furnishing a death certificate. This letter and the upcoming proposal to Parliament indicated that despite the advancement of medical theory in relation to diagnosing death, problems still existed when it came to its verification.

The continued evolution of the signs of death and regulation of the burial process caused the tests for death to evolve as well. The medical community was no longer reliant on cutting a vein to test for blood flow, or tickling the nostrils or throat to elicit a respiratory response. These new tests evolved from the theories of the anatomical and physiological understanding gained during the nineteenth century. Even during this late period, people were still being misdiagnosed as dead. During the middle of the nineteenth century, the cardiac and arterial failure test had gained in popularity. This test monitored the person's heartbeat for one to two minutes. If no cardiac sounds or movements were detected during this time, the person was assumed to be dead. However, this test for death was short lived because several people revived after having been declared as dead after using this method.

In 1896, William Tebb republished an article from the *Lancet* medical journal (1893), which promoted the use of the diaphanous test. During this test, the hand of the apparently dead person would be opened with the extended fingers just barely touching each other. The hand would then be held in front of a "strong artificial light" like the light bulb that Edison had patented less than fifteen years earlier.[31] The medical professional validating the person's death status would observe the space between the fingers. If a scarlet colored line appeared between each finger, it indicated that circulation was still in action. However, if no scarlet color was present, it indicated that circulation had ceased and the person had died. Another test for circulation was Monteverdi's Test, also called the ammonia blush test. During this test, the patient would be given a subcutaneous shot of ammonia to see if the area around the insertion point reddened. The red was the blood rushing to the surface and would prove the flow of blood. Despite the scientific nature of these tests, just like the centuries before, the only definitive way to ensure that the person was absolutely dead was to wait to see if the body putrefied over the course of a week.

In addition to the medical advancements of the nineteenth century, countries across Europe also started to officially enact funeral and burial laws. Typically these laws included the roles of physicians, medical examiners, and coroners. They also mandated the length of time that bodies needed to be kept before they could be buried. The role of the searcher, which had been so important during the plague of the seventeenth century, had been absorbed into the role of a registered medical practitioner or coroner. By 1893, the death certificate could be obtained from the coroner's office. Autopsies—then called post-mortem examinations—were used to validate the coroner's findings and to assure that the body had passed the point where it could be resuscitated.[32] Even as the twentieth century approached, the only other way to determine this absolute death was still waiting for the body to decay.

One of the most famous coroners in popular culture was from Munchkin Land in the 1939 movie *The Wizard of Oz*. He entered the narrative after Dorothy's house landed on the Wicked Witch of the West. While Dorothy was being indoctrinated into the idiosyncrasies of this strange new land, Oz, the coroner, entered the scene with the mayor and his advisors. The audience became aware of his position in Munchkin Land as the group discussed the importance of the witch being "morally, ethically, spiritually, physically, positively, undeniably, and reliably dead."[33] Holding up the "Certificate of Death" he proclaimed, "As coroner I must aver, I thoroughly examined her. And she's not only merely dead, she's really most sincerely dead."[34]

CHAPTER 8

The Restless Dead

"Advanced in years, Joseph Belk, of Lincoln. After he had been laid out for several hours, to all appearance dead, he raised himself up, and called for some tea to drink. His wife, who was then in the room with two or three neighbours, immediately ran out affrighted, but soon returned, and gave him what he wanted, which having drunk, he fell backward, and expired immediately."[1]

* * *

Folklorists have long debated the historic existence of the vampire throughout Europe and around the world. Historically, in Europe, vampires have been understood to be "people"—mythical or otherwise—whose survival was dependent on the ingestion of blood of the living. The ethnographer and folklorist Arnold van Gennep's theory on the Rites of Passage stated that there were rites that accompanied "every change of place, state, social position, and age."[2] The twentieth-century anthropologist Victor Turner expanded on this work by focusing on a transitional phase called "liminality." He explained that "liminal *personae*" or "threshold people" ambiguously transitioned through the stages of and sometimes became stuck "betwixt and between" the expected social or cultural norms.[3] If a threshold person became stuck between the stages of life and death, they would be alive but appear to be unconscious and unmoving, thereby giving the impression that they were trapped in a prolonged state of apparent death. Conversely, if a threshold person became stuck between the stages of death and life, they would have been touched by death but still have animated functions. People in this threshold space may have been identified as a revenant or vampire. They were not trusted and were considered to be dangerous and, in some cases, poisonous, contagious, or deadly. These perceptions caused them to be outcast from their communities and society in general. Fears relating to premature burial and people returning from the grave caused a general thrum of anxiety which coursed through the community as it considered how to respond to an encounter with someone who was neither alive nor dead. These anxieties were projected onto those believed to be vampires, blaming them for outbreaks of disease, such as plague, and for the unexplained deaths of people and livestock.[4]

In modern scholarship, vampires are typically considered as "an attempt by people of pre-industrial societies to explain the natural, but to them inexplicable, process of death and decomposition of the body."[5] The process of death was poorly understood through the Renaissance and then actively studied during the eighteenth and nineteenth centuries. Throughout that time, the medical community focused on keeping living people from being buried alive. In cases where people were accidentally buried alive, the focus of reports in books, newspapers, and pamphlets was on the state of the body when it was exhumed. When the coffin of an absolutely dead person was opened, textual evidence indicates that onlookers were startled to see how little corpses had decomposed. Folklorists and archeologists have discussed such common characteristics, such as reports that the blood inside the corpse flowed as though the person was still alive. The misconception that the corpse's hair and nails continued to grow after the corpse had been buried was caused by the tightening of the skin around the fingernails and scalp. Traditionally, vampires wore shrouds, indicating that they had been poor when they were alive. Their bodies were described as bloated, with a "ruddy or dark countenance."[6] It is plausible that this description came about because the person was suffering from hypoxia. The lack of oxygen inhaled by the person would have caused their fingers, toes, and areas around their mouth to take on a bluish gray hue and made the surrounding areas turn a more vibrant red. If a person had been prematurely buried, and were able to escape their grave, they may have returned in their burial shroud, bluish gray, with vibrant red lips and hands. Additionally, if they had been buried in a shallow grave or were buried towards the top of a mass grave, it is possible that the "ruddy" coloring could have come from the dirt that they would have climbed through while freeing themselves from their not-quite-final resting place. This would be especially plausible in locations with heavy soil, where it frequently rained, or the ground had a high clay content. Therefore, it is possible that those who came back from the grave and were deemed vampires could actually have been people who were misdiagnosed as dead, prematurely buried, and came back from the grave.

People did not typically know when a person who was being buried was going to become a vampire. However, those who suffered sudden deaths or were unable to put their end-of-life affairs in order were thought to be more likely to return from the dead than those who were able to properly plan for it. It was also believed that those who had been killed by outside forces were more likely to become revenants (people who came back from the dead) or vampires. Most stories of vampires do not explore the liminality of the person or when precisely they transitioned from human to monster. Nor do these stories consider the medical or public perspectives as those communities grappled to understand how the transition from life to death definitively concluded.

Along with various treatises on ghosts, spirits, and vampires, which were published prior to and throughout the Enlightenment and Romantic eras, literature began to echo these societal issues and related fears. The nineteenth century ushered in literature designed to both enhance and relieve fears of premature burial and the repercussions that followed. Authors during this era made the topic of premature burial more accessible by applying it to fiction. The medical community was still not completely certain about why people continued to be misdiagnosed as dead. Vampire fiction supplied reasons why it *might* have been happening. It also taught people about the signs of life and death in a way that kept readers coming back for more. On the surface, vampires appeared to be folklore whose link with the macabre and the mysterious had evolved similarly in different locales. However, the fictionalized stories included medical knowledge of the signs and symptoms of death as it was understood during the authors' times.

Popular culture has drawn a specific picture of a vampire. Dressed to the height of fashion, with pale skin and sharp, piercing eyes, with fangs, glistening in the moonlight they stalk their prey to drink the blood necessary to live through another night. Pale and often thin, these vampires sleep in coffins in order to protect themselves from the burning rays of the sun. Familiar though this image is, the description and characteristics of a vampire evolved over time. During the eighteenth century, vampires were considered to be walking or reanimated corpses. Often malevolent, they were known for causing the deaths of those whom they came in contact with. Their malevolence could take the form of outright murder, or bringing disease back to their homes and villages, or sucking the blood out of living people. By the nineteenth century, the concept of the vampire began to evolve with depictions in literature. And then, as things often do, the literature began to evolve and each story built upon those that came before it until, finally, it resembled the vampire genre of modern day horror.

Most historical accounts of vampires consisted of five common traits. The first was the reanimation of an apparently dead corpse. Then, the corpse then returned from the grave (2) and interacted with the living (3). Those interactions resulted in negative consequences, such as the spread of disease or people dying from blood depletion (4). Finally, the vampire returned to the grave (5). These factors were often echoed in vampire literature, with a particular focus on the reanimated corpse sucking the blood out of the living before returning to their coffin. However, vampire fiction often took liberties with these historical traits.

Literature which capitalized on fears of premature burial and/or the eternal worldly life after death included Samuel Coleridge's *Christabel* (1798, 1800), Robert Southey's *Thalaba the Destroyer* (1801), Lord Byron's *A Fragment of a Turkish Tale* (1813), and Polidori's prose *The Vampyre* (1819). These stories combined medical theories of the eighteenth and nineteenth centuries as they related to the signs and symptoms of death and resulted in medically-based supernatural stories that pushed the boundaries of known science. These early works of vampire fiction were written at the cusp of a medical evolution, just as modern medicine was about to shake off the superstitions of the past. However, the medical understanding and superstitions of the time were reflected in these examples of early vampire fiction. And, of course, what analysis of vampire literature against the medicine of the past would be complete without the inclusion of Bram Stoker's *Dracula*?

By the time Stoker's *Dracula* (1897) was written, nearly a century later, a whole new era of medicine had begun. Not representative of the earlier understanding of medicine and death, by the time *Dracula* was written, the concept and survivor experience of premature burial, which had terrified people for nearly two thousand years had fallen into the realm of superstition and lore. Armed with new technologies such as the binaural stethoscope (1852), a provable, viable germ theory (1860s), the application of that germ theory to prevent surgical infections (1867) and x-rays (1890s), physicians and surgeons of the late nineteenth century no longer identified with the more primitive conditions faced by the medical practitioners who came before.

The following analyses were not written to be all encompassing analytical reviews of vampire literature. Rather, they were chosen to provide context for how historical vampire stories, vampire literature, and the supporting medical theories are related. Each story was reviewed in context and compared against the five traits of historical vampire accounts from the preceding centuries. That said, not every metaphysical curiosity that was recorded in historical accounts can be easily or scientifically explained.

During the seventh century, for example, St. Cuthbert, the Bishop of Lindisfarne (England) (635 CE–687 CE), foresaw his own death and asked to be buried on the island of Inner Farne. The monks pleaded for his body to be buried at Lindisfarne instead, a right which he acquiesced before his death. Eleven years after his death, it was planned for his body to be exhumed for a ceremony at which the monks were going to proclaim his sainthood. The monks planned to display his skeleton to the celebrating crowds. Upon exhuming his body, however, they discovered that he had not decayed. Instead of being reduced to bones, his body looked as though it had been freshly buried. This peculiarity was taken as sign that he was, indeed, a saint. His body was redressed and interred in an aboveground tomb.

When the monastery was attacked by Vikings in 857 CE, the monks abandoned the site and resettled in the town of Chester-le-Street, England, until finally settling in Durham, England, in 995 CE—all the while carrying the tomb of St. Cuthbert with them. After the Norman Conquest in 1066, Benedictine monks took over the monastery in Durham. When the Benedictine Church was completed in 1104, St. Cuthbert was moved once again. When the legend of his uncorrupted body was questioned, the tomb was opened. Again, the body was said to have been whole, without decay, and not in the least skeletal. The body was re-entombed then enshrined during the Middle Ages, until the monastery dissolved during the Reformation. St. Cuthbert's body was moved again and secretly buried in a plain grave with goods such as "a gold and garnet pectoral cross, an ivory comb, a silver-covered portable altar, and a range of silks and embroidered vestments."[7] In 1827, his body was exhumed yet again. This time, however, only a skeleton and the grave goods remained. They were reburied and remained untouched until 1899 when a post-mortem review of the remains confirmed the high likelihood that it was the body of St. Cuthbert.

Definitions of a vampire varied between European countries and, in some cases, between regions within those countries. In addition to the five traits of a historical vampire story—with the exception of the earliest vampiric descriptions—the bodies of most vampires did not decompose. The bodies of vampires remained supple, without muscular atrophy, and were primed for life, even though they had been diagnosed as dead and their bodies disposed of up to years before they were seen again. Despite the regularity of these traits, vampire fiction did not necessarily include them all. The most important parallels of the fictional stories with the historical accounts were that the corpse reanimated and interacted with the living and that the story mentioned blood or transference of the life force in some way, generally relating to the vampire ingesting it. Therefore, while the story of St. Cuthbert's body is worthy of note, it was not a depiction of a vampire. St. Cuthbert's story was missing several identifiers that would have indicated an account of vampirism. He did not come back to life, break out of his grave, interact with the living, or drink their blood/take on their life force to regenerate his life.

One of the oldest vampire stories in Western Europe came from Celtic Ireland between the fifth and sixth centuries CE. During that time,

Ireland was divided into sections, each of which were independently ruled by chieftains. According to legend, the chieftain who was responsible for part of the northern Derry area was named Abhartach. He was believed to be a very short and tyrannical wizard. Those who he ruled over feared him and wanted to displace him from his seat of power. However, unseating or killing a chieftain was not easily done. So his subjects convinced another chieftain, named Cathán, to do it for them. After his murder, Abhartach was buried in a standing position in an isolated grave.

Abhartach returned from the grave the day after his funeral. His cruelty had not abated from the events of the night before. He demanded that "each person cut their wrist and bleed into his bowl daily in order to sustain his life."[8] Here we see the connection between blood and life over a millennium prior to the theories of William Harvey. When a second attempt to kill Abhartach ended with the same result, Cathán went to the Christian saint John (or Eoghan) for counsel. After listening to the story about the challenges faced while trying to permanently kill Abhartach, St. John explained that the evil chieftain was a practitioner of the dark arts and had "become one of the *neamh-mhairbh* [the undead]" as well as "a *dearg-diúlaí*, a drinker of human blood," which was the reason that he could not be killed or stay buried.[9] St. John suggested that Cathán try to restrain Abhartach and to kill him with a sword made of yew wood. The body was to be buried upside-down surrounded by ash twigs, with a heavy stone placed over the grave. Burying the body upside down would ensure that if Abhartach attempted to climb out of the grave, he would only dig himself deeper. The boulder would prevent Abhartach from escaping the grave if he found a way to turn himself around. St. John cautioned, however, that if the boulder was removed, Abhartach would be able to rise from the earth.

Cathán followed the instructions set forth by St. John. However, the sword made of yew only injured Abhartach. He was buried alive, headfirst to simulate being buried upside-down. Once the grave had been filled, it was "covered with ash branches, thorns, and a large boulder."[10] A stone monument was erected at the site. Now, a twisted tree grows sequestered off in the Glenullin area of County Derry, in the small town of Slaughtaverty. Large rocks lay beneath it, remains of the monument that once stood to commemorate a place that had been rife with fear and blood.

This incredible story included all the signs of vampirism. First, Abhartach's reanimated corpse returned from the grave and interacted with the living in a way that had negative consequences. Although Abhartach did not use the stereotypical fangs to drink the life force, he did demand that blood be given to him to drink. Finally, he returned to the grave—albeit against his will—but continued to return to the world of the living until he was forced to stay in his grave.

In many ways, it would be easy to assume that vampire stories were all folklore, superstition, or early fiction, where the monster was larger than life, a story told around the fire at night, featuring common people being brave in the face of inexplicable dangers. However, modern interpretations are less relevant than the contemporary experiences and beliefs which anchored these stories. Over the last 50 years, several archeological excavations have unearthed possible vampire burials, indicating that there was both awareness and concern in different communities. These burials were from as far back as the Middle Ages and included the physical aspects that indicated that the people buried had been recognized as vampires and had been dealt with accordingly.

One such grave dated back to the thirteenth century and was discovered at Perperikon, Bulgaria, in 2014. The skeletal remains were of a male who was approximately 45 years old. A two pound iron ploughshare had been hammered through his chest so hard that it broke his scapula and effectively pinned the corpse to the earth. The left leg of the corpse had also been disconnected and placed alongside the body. The excavator, Nikolay Ovcharov, was certain that they had discovered "an anti-vampire ritual."[11] The goal of such actions was to restrict the movement of the corpse of someone considered to be an evil, dangerous, or ungodly person, so that they could not rise from the grave and disturb the living.

Another vampire burial was found in 1994 on the far western island of Lesbos in Greece, which is situated just off the eastern coast of Turkey. In this case, the body was of a Muslim male who was buried in a wooden coffin in the wall of a crypt. The body had a stake running through the torso and "several heavy eight-inch-long iron spikes driven through the neck, pelvis and ankles, which pinned it down."[12] In his "Time to Slay Vampire Burials?" (2014) Dr. David Barrowclough asserted that this was "the only example of a non–Christian corpse to have been found treated in this fashion."[13] The reason that this corpse had been identified as a vampire has been lost to history, but it has been assumed that it may have been because he was an outsider from the community and therefore suspect.

While most historical vampire reports were of men, an apparent female vampire burial was discovered in 2006 on the island of Lazaretto Nuovo, near Venice, Italy. The corpse was found in a sixteenth-century mass burial pit filled with the remains of plague victims. Her jaw had been wrenched open and a brick was shoved into the mouth. The forensic archeologist, Matteo Borrini, in conjunction with the University of Florence (Italy), collaborated with a team of scientists to discover what they could about the remains of the female vampire. It was determined that she was from Europe and died in her sixties. She ate a diet high in grains and vegetables, denoting that she was likely lower class.[14] Due to her advanced age, some scholars have mused that she may have been considered a witch rather than a vampire. However, the brick placed in her mouth to dislocate her jaw, thus making it impossible for her to chew through her burial shroud and escape her grave indicated fears of vampirism rather than witchcraft.

During the twelfth century, William of Newburgh (1136–1198) chronicled "a history of memorable events" that had occurred in England in his *Historia rerum Anglicarum*.[15] He claimed that "undead corpses" were plentiful during the early Middle Ages, especially in England. According to Newburgh, one such undead corpse tormented the inhabitants of Anantis Castle, which is currently thought to be Alnwick Castle in Northumberland. The being that wandered around within the castle walls during the night smelled like a rotting corpse. Those who caught a whiff of his foul stench were said to have contracted the plague.[16] In order to protect themselves, the inhabitants of the castle shut themselves inside their private dwellings and did not go out after dark because they believed that they were safer in the daylight.

Those living in the castle appealed to the town leaders for assistance. When a resolution took too long, two brothers whose father had died of the plague decided to take the issue into their own hands. They went to the cemetery and dug up the corpse's shallow grave. They discovered the corpse laying in the grave, its shroud torn to tatters and the body so gorged on blood that it was described as being "swollen to an enormous corpulence."[17] They struck the body with a spade and so much blood came out of it that the body was compared to a leech that had been "filled with the blood of many persons."[18] There is some ambiguity about this description, however, and it seems to depend on the translation. There could have been a gush of blood as if the statement was meant to imply that the "undead corpse" had ingested a large quantity of blood. Another theory is that there was a trickle of blood because the body was filled with as much blood as an engorged leech. Either way when a body decomposes, the heart ceases to pump blood. Within four months the blood oxidizes and blackens as the iron from the blood vessels is released. While an airtight seal on a stone coffin could have prevented the corpse from decomposing, it would not have explained why blood still flowed throughout his body. Since a dead body naturally swells up as gases are released as part of the putrefaction process, it was possible that they observed this and misunderstood the source of the swelling and blood. In either case, there were concerns that the corpse would continue to reanimate.

Accordingly, a funeral pyre was built, and the body was laid upon it. The heart was removed from the corpse and the rest of the body was set on fire. Removing its heart ensured that the corpse would no longer return to life, and burning the body prevented future reanimation. After the corpse had been destroyed "the pestilence which was rife among the people ceased, as if the air, which had been corrupted by the contagious motions of the dreadful corpse, were already purified by the fire which had consumed it."[19] The use of the word "purified" is notable. During this time, the concept of purifying the body with fire may have been considered the first step to purify the soul so that it would be able to leave purgatory and be admitted into Heaven.

Newburgh's vampire story also fits the general expectations of a historical vampire story. Even though people in the Middle Ages thought that the soul was strong enough to reanimate a corpse, Newburgh believed that the devil animated the corpse and gave it the ability to rise out of the grave. Since the word "vampire" did not evolve into common vernacular until the eighteenth century, most stories prior to that used other words to describe the same phenomenon. Many used the word "revenant" to indicate someone who returned after dying. Newburgh used the term "undead corpse." This terminology gave the immediate impression that the body had reanimated post death. The tale of Newburgh's vampire as it roamed the halls of the castle trying to interact with the living indicated that the living feared and avoided this interaction. Arguably even more terrifying than a wandering, interactive, undead corpse was the fear of catching the plague from the odor.

The Life and Miracles of Virgin Saint Morwenna was also published in England during the twelfth century. The story combined supernatural elements with the signs of vampirism to create a story unlike the others. In it, two peasants moved from the town of Stapenhill, which was overseen by the Benedictine Monastery Burton Abbey, to the parish of Drakelow in South Derbyshire, which did not come under the purview of the abbey. When the abbey tried to extradite them, the knight who oversaw Drakelow refused to force them to return. In response, the monks prayed to St. Morwenna for help. The two men died abruptly the next day and were buried soon after. Whether or not they stayed dead for very long was open to interpretation, however, since that night they were both seen walking up the road "carrying their coffins on their backs."[20] Most people, in particular the peasantry, during this time were only wound in burial shrouds prior to being committed to the earth. So the detail that they had been seen carrying their coffins meant that they had been buried well, that they had not been buried at all and were only enclosed in their coffins, or it was a case of mistaken identity. Soon thereafter, rumors started circulating around Drakelow that the undead were haunting the town, in the form of an animal like a large dog or a bear. These animals could be heard beating upon the walls of people's homes, or, in some cases, calling for the inhabitants to come outside. As the town was besieged by these supernatural animals, an unspecified disease swept through the area and decimated most of the town's population. That caused the bodies of the two peasants be exhumed. Both peasants who had supposedly been seen walking down the road with their coffins on their backs were found buried in their graves inside their coffins.

As with most historical vampire stories, their bodies had not decayed and their burial shrouds were bloodied, especially around their faces. In response, their corpses were beheaded, and the heads were put in between their legs. Then their hearts were removed from their chests and burned. The remains were put back into their coffins, which were nailed shut again before dirt was shoveled back on top of them. Similar to Newburgh's story, the disease outbreak ceased immediately after the peasants' bodies were decapitated and reinterred. Despite the cessation of the disease, the remaining inhabitants abandoned the town. Literature of the late eighteenth century and through the nineteenth century was based, in part from historical vampire stories such as the vampires of Anantis Castle and Drakelow. Winding in tales from the historical vampire accounts, authors used the history of medicine and recent history to engage with the public.

Samuel Coleridge's (1772–1834) gothic poem *Christabel* was written during the late eighteenth century. There is some debate over when the first part was written, either in 1797 or 1798. It is known that Coleridge wrote the first part of this poem while he was at Stowey, which is where he was staying at the cusp of January to February in 1798. He, his friend William Wordsworth, and William's sister Dorothy spent many days enjoying their natural surroundings. Dorothy journaled about their time together and wrote fondly of the nature around them. Some similar phrasing was used in *Christabel*, so it is likely that the first part of the poem was written in 1798. The second part of *Christabel* was written in 1800 while Coleridge resided in Keswick, England. Although their time together was shorter, Coleridge visited with William and Dorothy for a few weeks on his way to Keswick. He had been suffering from writer's block and had trouble completing the poem. But after a night of imbibing heavily at the house of a local clergyman, the fog lifted and his "verse-making faculties returned."[21] The final 20 lines of the second part were not included in the surviving copies of the poem, nor was it included in an early transcription (circa 1801–1815) by Sarah Hutchinson (the future Mrs. William Wordsworth). Instead, he sent the final part to his friend Robert Southey.

Most theories that connect the poem *Christabel* to vampirism showcase the theme of the sexually alluring, "half-mythical, half-pathological conception of the witch."[22] This is illustrated by the antagonist of the poem: Geraldine. In contrast to the innocent, pious and kind maiden, Christabel,

Geraldine is strong, regal, and mature. Under the guise of familiarity, she befriends Christabel and uses magic to bewitch her. Ever the good hostess, Christabel invites Geraldine into the home that she shares with her father. By the time she realizes that Geraldine is not a kind person, she is too far under her spell to stop the events which Geraldine had set into motion. By the time she was able to discuss the situation with her father, she was not believed. At the end of the poem, Geraldine transforms herself to look like Christabel's absent fiancé. Although she went through the motions of being dutifully betrothed, Christabel could tell that something was wrong … that her fiancé was not who he appeared to be. Despite the distance growing between them, she and the transformed Geraldine approach the altar to be wed. At the last possible moment, her real fiancé arrives and shows her a ring that she had given him before he went away. Once the deception is realized, Geraldine disappears. In the end, Christabel married her correct suitor.

Throughout *Christabel*, there is hardly a word about anatomy, physiology, life or death, save the explanation of Christabel's mother, who had died during childbirth. The nature of Geraldine is not explained in great detail, except that she was a witch or a demon who was capable of doing actual magic, such as casting glamours on herself to change her appearance. She bound Christabel with enchantments to make her seem to forget her real fiancé. Geraldine did not fit the criteria necessary to be identified as a historical vampire. However, there were parts of her character that transformed the reader's expectations of a vampire in popular culture. "Don't ever invite a vampire into your house, you silly boy. It renders you powerless."[23]

After encountering Geraldine in the woods, Christabel invited her to come home with her. She warns that her father is in ill health and to be quiet as they walk through the castle. In this section, we see that Geraldine was not able to cross the threshold into the household without the necessary permissions transferred as Christabel carried Geraldine through the gate.

> They crossed the moat, and Christabel
> Took the key that fitted well;
> A little door she opened straight,
> All in the middle of the gate;
> The gate that was ironed within and without,
> Where an army in battle array had marched out.
> The lady sank, belike through pain,
> And Christabel with might and main
> Lifted her up, a weary weight,
> Over the threshold of the gate:
> Then the lady arose again,
> And moved, as she were not in pain.[24]

After granting Geraldine tacit permission to enter her home, Christabel slowly lost her ability to think for herself and fell deeper and deeper under Geraldine's spell. A footnote in Earnest Hartley Coleridge's collected works of *Christabel by Samuel Taylor Coleridge* (1907) stated, "No demon could without aid pass the holy emblem over the lintel. There is a profound moral in this popular superstition. The devil cannot come into a house unless you bring him in yourself."[25] This is not to say that witches are demons, only that malevolent beings, by any name, could not cross the threshold of someone's home without permission from those who lived there.

When compared against the list of traits which were identified in historic vampire stories, *Christabel* does not fit. However, when compared to other stories about female vampires, the element of dangerous allure becomes evident. The theme of the female seductress or the femme fatale has been repeated as a literary trope. It predates the Romantic era and has its roots in mythology, such as the myth of Lilith. In his book *The Living Dead: A Study of the Vampire in Romantic Literature* (1981), James B. Twitchell described Lilith as "the Hebraic temptress who supposedly turned to blood-sucking after being spurned by Adam."[26] The female seductress also inspired J. Sheridan Le Fanu's vampire-erotic tale, *Carmilla* (1872). Coleridge's literary vampire, Geraldine, exemplified this alluring and erotic femme fatale.

Situations regarding people being stuck in the liminal phase were reported throughout history. They may have appeared as femmes fatale, disease carrying reanimated corpses, or blood-sucking monsters. A story from thirteenth-century Gascony explored the belief that death did not occur immediately when the soul was separated from the body. Instead it implied that the body could possibly live without the soul. As recounted, a priest sprinkled holy water over the graves in the cemetery surrounding his church as he prayed for the souls of the dead. He continued to do this until one day the dead rose up from their graves and held out their hands in supplication for more holy water. Like Newburgh's vampire, the priest saw people physically rise from their graves. In contrast to Newburgh's vampire, however, those who rose out of the grave in Gascony were not harmful. They merely requested more holy water, as though they were thirsty before returning to their graves.[27] Keeping in line with the five traits of a vampire story, these souls reanimated, rose from the grave, interacted with the living, and returned to the grave. Rather than drinking blood, they drank water … something necessary for bodily survival.

During the late seventeenth and early eighteenth centuries reports came out of Central Europe claiming that the dead were not staying dead or buried. Beyond the concept of being misdiagnosed as dead, these reports included the actions taken by the no-longer-apparently dead. There were reports of the once-dead walking, interacting with their surroundings, abusing or injuring both people and animals, and sucking the blood of their close family.[28] It was believed that these actions, especially the latter, caused the failing health and death of those whose blood had been sucked out. Once a community identified that a vampire was in their midst, steps were taken to protect the living and make sure that the dead remained so.

In 1655, the British philosopher Henry More (1614–1687) attempted to use rational, empirical evidence to prove the existence of vampires and witches and to include them in a "universal order" ranging from God to atheists.[29] His *Antidote Against Atheism* (1653) relayed the story of a shoemaker in Breslau, Poland. This shoemaker had committed self-murder (suicide) by cutting his own throat on September 20, 1591. Lutheranism was generally practiced in the area and did not rely on the necessity of the body being buried in consecrated ground in order for the soul to be admitted into Heaven. Nonetheless, his wife wanted him to be buried in the churchyard, so she hid the wound within the folds of the burial shroud. Since he had lived a good life, and nobody had any reason to doubt his wife's assertion that he had died from a stroke, the local pastor allowed him to be buried in the churchyard.

A little over a month later, rumors began circulating about the cause of his death and his wife was named in an inquiry. Despite her sticking to her story that he had died of natural causes, people doubted her claims. As the inquest continued, people started to report that they were seeing the shoemaker in their dreams and as they awoke in the early morning. The nightmarish visions were tame in comparison to the waking dreams that were being experienced by other people in the community. Several people reported that the shoemaker appeared lying near them in their beds. They felt as though he was committing acts of violence against them, such as pressing on them, hitting them, or pinching them until they bruised. Some even reported that "impressions of his fingers would be upon sundry parts of their bodies in the mornings."[30] When these occurrences continued through the winter, the authorities decided that actions needed to be taken to stop them.

The shoemaker's body was disinterred in April 1592, eight months after he had been laid to rest. As with other stories of vampires, the body had not putrefied at all. The only musty smell came from the burial clothes. His limbs and joints were flexible, and his skin was fresh, although it hung loosely upon his body. The wound on his neck remained open and had neither corrupted nor healed. Unlike most vampire stories, the authorities did not cause immediate harm to the body. Instead, they disinterred it and put it on public display so that it could be watched at all times for signs of life. Since the signs of life and death were still ambiguous during the late sixteenth century, the disinterment and subsequent watching of the body indicated suspicions that he may have still been alive.

Even as the body was being watched, the townspeople continued to be tormented in both their dreams and during their waking hours. In response, the shoemaker was buried under the town's gallows. A month later, the dreams and torments continued, so the corpse was disinterred again. This time, it was noticed that the body appeared to have grown fatter, and the alarmed community responded accordingly. Not only did they behead the corpse, but its legs and arms were also detached. They removed the heart, through the back of the corpse, before burning the body. The heart, they noted, "was as fresh and entire as in a calf newly killed."[31]

The story of the shoemaker was different from the other historical stories mentioned because it included some supernatural elements. This vampire's interactions were much more personal than they had been in prior reports. Rather than physically seeing the appearance of a ghost or having physical interactions with an undead corpse, the deceased appeared in peoples' psyche while they were both asleep and awake. These visions included the intimacy of the vampire winding up in their bed with them and placing its hands on people in unnamed private areas. In response, there were additional retaliatory actions taken against the shoemaker's body. They removed the corpse's brain (head) and heart, as well as the lungs since they entered the body through the back. They also disjointed the body so extensively that if it reanimated, it would not be able to use its head, arms, or legs, even prior to lighting the body on fire. Once the body was mutilated and destroyed, the townspeople's nightmares and visions ended.

Commonly, in the historical reporting of vampires, writers maintained that reburying a corpse would stop troublesome apparitions from appearing. During the fourteenth century, for example, Richard Fitzalan, the Earl of Arundel (1346–1397) had a habit of antagonizing and opposing King Richard II (1367–1400). In response, the King had Fitzalan arrested and beheaded. Rumors began circulating that the Earl's body had been reunited with his head. After hearing the rumors, King Richard II began to have nightmares, seeing the Earl's ghost flickering before him and threatening him with "indescribable terrors."[32] Haunted by these nightmares, the King ordered that Fitzalan be exhumed. Although the nobles who exhumed the body refuted the rumors and stated that the body and head had not been reunited, King Richard II was still unnerved. To ensure that Fitzalan's head and body would not be reunited, the King requested that the signs indicating where the Earl had been buried be removed and the body be reburied under the floor of an Augustinian church.

Reports of vampires made their way out of Poland in 1693–1694. In these stories "oupires," loosely translated to "vampires or ghosts," appeared in the afternoon and evening.[33] They ate the linen that was wrapped around their bodies and came out of their graves. The oupires then became malicious and violently hugged their family or friends, wrapping their arms around them like a python, and gorging themselves on the victim's blood until they were utterly sated. Overeating resulted in blood flowing from the oupire's nose and ears. In more extreme cases the corpse swam in blood as it "'oozed' out of the coffin."[34] The only way to stop these murders was to behead the oupires or "open the heart of the ghost" in cases where the heart inside the body was still supple and pliable, like that of a living person.[35] After the blood was released from the oupire's body, it was sometimes made into bread. It was believed that those who ate the bread would be protected from the spirit that no longer reanimated the corpse.

Stories of "certain dead Bodies (called here Vampyres) [that] had killed several Persons by sucking out all of their Blood" made their way into the British press during the early eighteenth century.[36] The *Country Journal, or the Craftsman* (1732), *Whitehall's Evening Post* (1733), and *Applebee's Original Weekly Journal* (1733) printed a story of the Serbian hajduk, Arnold Paul, which had taken place five years earlier. A hajduk was an outlaw fighter who defended their home from the rule of the Habsburgs (German) or the Ottoman Empire (Turkish). Throughout his life, Paul had told stories of being "tormented" by a "vampyre" near the town of Caschaw in Lower Hungary and near the border of Turkish Serbia.[37] In an attempt to rid himself of its attention, he ate some dirt from the vampire's grave and "rubbed himself with their Blood."[38] About a month after his death, his neighbors started complaining that he had returned and was killing people. When his body was exhumed forty days later, it was noticed that he had not decomposed. Not only that, but fresh, bright, blood was coming out of his nose, mouth, and ears, covering his burial shroud and winding sheet. Finally, his fingernails and toenails had fallen out and new ones had grown in. Upon seeing these signs it was decided that he had become a vampire and needed to be dealt with. He groaned when the stake was driven through his heart and blood poured from his chest. His corpse was then burned, and his ashes buried in his grave. Paul's reanimation perpetuated the community's belief that people whose lives were tormented or ended by vampires then became vampires after their own deaths. Therefore, the corpses of several other people who were associated with vampires were staked and burned and the remains reburied.

Historically, stories of the supernatural have received attention from those who would like to present a plausibly simple explanation. During the early eighteenth century, Serbia was torn between the Ottoman and

Habsburg empires and was "subject to the whims of two competing super-powers."[39] Therefore, it is sometimes theorized that the increase of reports of vampires, or undead corpses, stemmed from an unconscious desire for Serbians to assert "their own agency on the world."[40] The story of Arnold Paul, sometimes spelled Paole, is one of the most infamous stories of vampirism during the eighteenth century. The article that recounted the Arnold Paul story in the *Country Journal, or the Craftsman* (1732) included an alternative theory about how vampires could exist without corpses reanimating. The article was organized as a conversation between the author, a physician and a "*beautiful young Lady*, who was a great Admirer of *strange* and *wonderful Occurrences*."[41] The author, Nicholas Amhurst (1697–1742), pen-named Caleb D'Anvers, was the only conversationalist identified. D'Anvers was the editor of the paper, and he provided a political perspective on the vampire narrative. The physician considered vampire stories to be fictional because they challenged what he knew about death. The young lady approached the conversation from a more literal perspective and believed that the story of Arnold Paul was true because the time, places, and names of the affected and those who performed the investigation were stated. She also pointed out that the official report appeared to have been sent to the Court of Vienna where it was verified by six surgeons and two officers from the Army, whom she believed to be subject matter experts.

Despite the evidence that was pointed out by the young lady, the physician was not swayed. Confident in the medical theory of the time, he posited that the opinions of those who had not studied medicine would not have the knowledge to convince him that "a *dead Body* whose animal Powers were totally extinguish'd could torment the living by *sucking their Blood* or performing any other *active and operative Functions*."[42] This discussion took place before the resuscitative process was created, before Winslow was able to remind the medical community that people were being misdiagnosed as dead, and before the definition of death was understood to be inadequate. But the young lady was not as easily convinced and reminded the physician that there were other outrageous theories that the medical community *had* believed and encouraged others to believe in as well before they were disproven. She mused that perhaps this situation fell into the same category.

After the physician and the young woman came to an impasse, D'Anvers presented an alternative theory on the vampire debate. Although he agreed that a dead body could not perform any functions of life, he still believed that the dead could torment the living. Since the Hungarians had spent a considerable amount of time being ruled by other countries, they were in a precarious situation when it came to airing grievances. As a result, any complaints tended to be written in an allegorical style. Because of this, he believed that the story of Arnold Paul, specifically, and general stories of vampires from that area of Europe, were satirical ways for people to complain about their political situation. For example, the concept of a vampire sucking the blood out of people in their community may have been a way of secretly accusing an oppressive ministry of benefiting from violence, taxes, and fattening themselves on "the Vitals of his Country."[43] This oppression could have also tormented the living and continued from beyond the grave because people had to mortgage or sell their homes and land to pay their taxes. It would be folly to think that they would become part of the ministry if they paid enough taxes. Instead, he asserted, that the sale of people's property gutted any inheritance that may have been passed on to their next generation, which left their descendants at a disadvantage.

This perspective can be applied to the story of Arnold Paul. Paul's dissatisfaction with the current regime was evidenced by his being a hajduk. D'Anvers explanation completely skipped the actions that Paul took to protect himself (eating dirt from the vampire's grave and rubbing himself with its blood), although he could have strengthened his argument by proposing that Paul was in league with the ministry, having eaten their food or been paid to work for them. D'Anvers believed that the actions of driving a stake through the heart and burning the body were ridiculous and fictitious ways to dissuade other people from adopting the unspecified "same practices" as Arnold Paul.[44] He also theorized that the blood that came out of Paul alluded to the "corrupt wages" that he "suck'd out of the Veins of his Countrymen."[45] Theft of this sort would have caused people do die due to pauperism rather than from blood loss.

D'Anvers also alluded to Descartes' theory of the separation of the body and the mind to explain why Paul's body did not decompose. Rather than allowing the word "corruption" to represent the putrefaction of the body, he decided that it referred to the wickedness of man, a personality trait found in the mind, which ceased to exist when the mind stopped working. Although D'Anvers pointed out the body and the mind were separate and that the personality lived in the mind, he did not discuss the effects of separating the body and the soul. Despite the article being written for the British public, there was no mention of the afterlife or the Judgment of God. D'Anvers merely postulated that his inability to explain the reasoning for the destruction of Paul's body proved that it was not true. He changed the subject and declared the entire story and stories like it to be

a *Fable* or *Fiction*, made use of to convey a satirical Invective against some living *Oppressor*; for as a *dead Corpse* cannot perform any *vital Functions* (according to the judicious Observation of my *learned Friend* there) so neither can it be sensible of any *Pain*, or express it by any *Sounds*, tho' a thousand Stakes should be driven through it.[46]

The story of Arnold Paul influenced vampire literature during the following century. Both Robert Southey (1774–1843) and Lord Byron (1788–1824) wrote stories that drew from the narrative of the buried dead returning home to torment the living. Southey's epic poem, *Thalaba the Destroyer*, was written between 1796 and 1800 and published in 1801. There is some debate over which story featured the first vampire in English fiction: *Christabel* or *Thalaba the Destroyer*. While *Christabel* utilized the character archetype of the femme fatale, *Thalaba the Destroyer* explored several superstitions relating to vampires, including many of the traits that were repeated in historic accounts of vampires.

Southey's *Thalaba the Destroyer* took place in Arabia. The protagonist, Thalaba was destined to go through various trials and tribulations to fight against the magic that sorcerers had cast upon his family. Several historians and literary theorists have written about the political and religious connections between Thalaba, his country, and England. Dr. Carol Bolton explained that the poem was "constructed in a way that discusses issues within British as well as Middle Eastern society."[47] Bolton noted that Thalaba "operates as a device to criticize his own society ... [and is perceived] as embodying ideal 'British' characteristics."[48] These "ideal characteristics" were also utilized when Southey described the body of Oneiza, Thalaba's deceased bride. Although Oneiza had died on their wedding day, Thalaba informed his father-in-law that he continued to see her at night. So, one rainy night, the two of them entered her underground tomb. As midnight crested the night, they saw a green glowing light spread throughout the tomb's chamber.

> And in that hideous light
> Oneiza stood before them. It was She,...
> Her very lineaments,... and such as death
> Had Changed them, livid cheeks, and lips of blue;
> But in her eyes there dwelt
> Brightness more terrible
> Than all the loathsomeness of death.
> "Still art thou living, wretch?"
> In hollow tones she cried to Thalaba;
> "And must I nightly leave my grave
> To tell these, still in vain,
> God hath abandon'd thee?"[49] [Book 8, verse 9].

In this poem, Oneiza literally rose from the dead. This was evidenced by the fact that she stood before her husband and father and admitted to leaving her grave on a nightly basis. Although her face looked the same as it did when she had died, the coloration had changed. Her cheeks are described as being livid, meaning that they were bright in color. However, her lips were blue, which is caused by a lack of oxygen. Because of these two contrasting visual cues, she appears to be a threshold person, stuck in a phase between death and life. The brightness in her eyes and her ability to speak indicated that the vital principle was still alive within her. Throughout this explanation, four of the five criteria of a historical vampire story were satisfied: the reanimated corpse, coming out of the grave, returning to her loved one, and returning to the grave. The only missing criteria was that she did not drink the blood or otherwise transfer living energy to herself while she was animated.

Not only did she look and act like a historical vampire, but she "died" like one too. Upon hearing her speak to Thalaba, her father exclaimed his disbelief that it was really hear speaking. Holding a lance out to Thalaba, he demanded that Thalaba strike down the corpse standing before them. When Thalaba could not bring himself to do so, his close friend, Moath, whom he did not realize had followed them down into the tomb, thrust a lance through Oneiza's body, causing her to howl as the forces that had lived within her body were driven out.

> When Moath, firm of heart,
> Perform'd the bidding: through the vampire corpse
> He thrust his lance; it fell,
> And howling with the wound,
> Its fiendish tenant fled[50] [Book 8, verse 10].

In addition to calling Oneiza's undead corpse a vampire, Southey also included extensive notes in the appendix in his book to validate this point. He included stories of vampirism that had been published throughout history. One such story was from 1736 Sclavonia (modern-day Slavonia). According to the story, three days after an old man was buried, he reappeared at home and asked his son for something to eat before he disappeared. Two days later, the old man returned. It was not recorded if the young man complied with his father's requests. However, the following morning the son was found "dead in his bed."[51] Soon after, people in the village started falling ill. After receiving word of the situation, the tribunal in Belgrade sent two commissioners and an executioner to the village to gather more information. Upon arriving at the village, they began to open the graves of people who had been buried for six weeks or less. When they came to the old man's grave, they found "his eyes open, his colour fresh, his respiration quick and strong, yet he appeared to be still and insensible."[52] They concluded that he was "a notorious *Vampire*."[53] In response, the executioner drove "a stake through his heart" and then placed the body in a bonfire, burning it to ash.[54]

Along with the familiar story of Arnold Paul, Southey also included a story from Greece from the end of 1700. The Grecian story told of a troublesome apparition whose body was disinterred and dissected ten days after it had been buried. The body had already begun to decay, and it stank so badly that frankincense was burned to try to mask the smell. Unfortunately, all it did was add to the stench in the church where the dissection took place. After a butcher removed the heart, it was decided that the best course of action was to burn it. Despite disinterment, dissection, and destruction of the heart, the apparition continued to return to the village, banging on doors, windows, and roofs. People left their homes and chose to camp near the edges of town in order to get away from it. Fearful, people sprinkled holy water around the town and used it to wash doors. People thrust the blades of swords down into the grave several times a day. The only thing that stopped the apparition from returning was the re-exhumation and total destruction of its body.

During the beginning of the nineteenth century, the poet Lord Byron was unimpressed with the Romantic style of poetry and much preferred the neoclassical style of the eighteenth and nineteenth centuries. An idealistic deist, Byron was introspective and aware of the world around him. Born to poor parents, Byron's birth name was George Gordon Byron. He was born with a clubbed foot, which his mother was just as likely to taunt him for as she was to find doctors to try to fix it.[55] When he was ten, he inherited the Baronial seat and became the sixth Baron Byron, the titled peerage of the Barony of Byron in England.

After moving to the residential seat, Byron's life changed considerably. Through his school years, he enjoyed writing speeches, poetry, and letters of correspondence. He achieved a Master of Arts at Trinity College, Cambridge, in 1808. While there, he began to favor liberalist politics and joined the Cambridge Whig Club. He left Trinity when the club's journal published a harsh critique about work that he had published anonymously. He attended his seat in the House of Lords after moving to London in 1809. While in London, he enjoyed an extravagant lifestyle and partook in many of the past-times that the city offered, such as fencing, boxing, attending the theater, and writing.

Byron continued to publish anonymously. His first major poetical work was titled *English Bards, and Scotch Reviewers. A Satire* (1809). This satirical work was aimed at many of the most notable poets and playwrights of the time, including Samuel Taylor Coleridge, Robert Southey, and William Wordsworth.[56] After his book was well-received, Byron felt vindicated and took time to travel to Greece. After a short, unfulfilling marriage, he moved to Geneva in 1816, where he became acquainted with Mary Godwin (1797–1851; later Mary Shelley) and her future husband

Percy Shelley. After 1817, Byron continued to tour through Europe, eventually returning to England in 1823 as a member of the London Committee. This committee had been created in order to assist in the Greeks' fight for independence from Turkey. Lord Byron was stricken by a fever and died a year later at the age of 36.

Throughout his short career, the tone of Byron's plays and poems often embodied his moods and interests at the time. This provided for a range of literary contributions that included any combination of idealism, humor, melancholy, cynicism, or realism. Among his many literary contributions, he was responsible for creating the now classic, haunted, melancholy, defiant hero.[57] Byron wrote *A Fragment of a Turkish Tale* in 1813, as he tried to balance two romantic relationships, neither of which concluded in his favor. The story is about Leila, a woman who in love with a Christian but enslaved to the Turkish lord Hassan. After her love interest was discovered, Hassan had her put into a sack and drowned in the ocean. In consequence, the Christian murdered Hassan but was so remorseful for his actions that he banished himself to a monastery.

Byron's inclusion of the vampire comes quite obviously in lines 755–762:

> But, first, on earth as Vampire sent,
> They corse [*sic*] shall from its tomb be rent;
> Then ghastly haunt thy native place,
> And suck the blood of all they race,
> There from thy daughter, sister, wife,
> At midnight drain the stream of life;
> Yet loathe the banquet which perforce
> Must feed thy living corse;
> Thy victims ere they yet expire
> Shall know the daemon for their sire,
> As cursing thee, thou cursing them,
> Thy flowers are wither'd on the stem....[58]

Through Byron's imagery, he identifies four of the five concepts of the historical vampire. He explains that the "living cor[p]se" would reanimate and rise up from the grave. Once the vampire returned, it interacted with the living by sucking their blood until they withered and died. The only concept of the historical vampire that is not mentioned in his poem is the return to the grave. Adding to the image of the vampire that would later become part of popular culture, Byron mentioned that the vampire sucks the blood out of the living in order to feed itself. After the publication of this book, this concept became one of the cornerstones of the literary vampire.

In the following passage, Byron also connected blood with life, showing at least a basic understanding of medical theory from the eighteenth century. This implied understanding continued in the same passage when Byron commented on how people looked when they were dying. The image of "her cheek's last tinge" referred to the way someone dying would look as the blood drained out of her body. Likewise, his inclusion of how the vital spark (soul) diminished in her eyes, causing them to become glassy as she died.

> Yet must though end they task, and mark
> Her cheek's last tinge, her eye's last spark,
> And the last glassy glance must view
> Which freezes o'er its lifeless blue[59];

* * *

Even while the medical community was making strides away from the humoral-based practices of the preceding era, there was still a fair amount of misunderstanding and superstition about life and death. During the mid-eighteenth century, Pope Benedict XIV (1675–1758) did his own research on "the lore of bodies corruptible and incorruptible" and declared that vampires were "the 'fallacious fictions of human fantasy.'"[60] Although the Pope had made his view on the matter of vampirism clear, information on vampires continued to be published in England and throughout Western Europe. *The Phantom World: The History and Philosophy of Spirits, and Vampires or Ghosts of Hungary, Moravia, etc.* (1751, translated 1851) was the culmination of over 50 years of research and is considered to be one of the "most in-depth, interrogative, and widely read vampire treatises of the era."[61] In this book, the French monk Augustin Calmet (1672–1757) set forth stories of angels, demons, ghosts, and vampires. Nearly half of the book focused on vampires: causes, stories, and ways to kill them, as proven in Eastern Europe. He discussed cases where bodies that had been buried for over a year still showed typical signs of life, such as "the blood in a liquid state, the flesh entire, the complexion fine and florid, [and] the limbs flexible and pliable."[62] Calmet also noticed that corpses of people who died from disease or poisoning looked similar to those that had been accused of vampirism; he identified that their blood bubbled and rarefied rather than congealing in their veins as expected.[63] Other signs of life that vampiric corpses continued to show included the continued growth of their hair and nails, rosy cheeks, and the appearance of weight gain.

One such vampire story was recorded as having taken place around 1730. A German soldier was lodged at the home of a Hungarian peasant and was surprised when a stranger came in and sat down at the table that he shared with his host. He noticed that his host seemed quite startled by this visitor. However, since the soldier was a guest and did not know the history between the two, he remained a passive observer. When the host died the following day, the soldier's curiosity got the better of him and he asked for details about what had happened the day before. He was informed that the stranger was the host's father, who had died and been buried for ten years, and that he had told his son that he was going to die. It was believed that not only had the no-longer-dead father come to visit, but he also caused the death of the son.[64]

When the soldier told his military regiment about what had occurred, they commissioned the Captain of the Alandetti infantry, the Count de Cabreras, to run an inquiry regarding the account. After taking sworn statements from the other people who lived in the house, the Count discovered that the soldier's story was accurate. Upon further inquiry, the people of the village corroborated the story. As the Count continued to collect evidence, the grave of the host's father was opened and those who were in attendance saw that the body had not decomposed and blood still ran through his veins. In response, the Count cut off the head of the host's father and set the body back inside.

The relayed account of the soldier has enough traits to be considered a historical vampire interaction. The host's father had been believed to be dead for over ten years. Yet, his body reanimated and came out of his tomb. Upon arriving at the family's home, he interacted with his son (the host) and foretold of his death which occurred that night. After his impromptu visit to his family, the father went back into his tomb. When exhumed, he resembled someone who had recently died, including the fluidity of the blood. These circumstances caused the Count de Cabreras to regard the story seriously and behead the body before allowing it to be reinterred.

As the Count gathered evidence relating to the soldier's story of the death caused by a mysterious visitor, he was made aware of other similar stories from the area. One was about a man who had been dead for over thirty years but had returned to his home three times. The visits were always around the time when the family gathered to eat. And he always came hungry. The first time, he "sucked the blood out of the neck of his own brother."[65] The second time that he returned, he sucked blood from his son. The third time that he returned, he sucked the blood from one of the servants. All three of the people who were fed upon died immediately. This story also had the relevant traits to be considered a historical vampire story. In this case, the apparently dead man had reanimated and gone back to his home three times. Rather than merely foretelling death, he caused it by sucking the blood out of his brother, his son, and the servant before returning to his grave.

The Count had the body of this vampiric offender exhumed as well. The blood in this body also resembled the fluidity of the blood of a living person. In response, the Count had "a large nail" driven through the man's temple before the body was reinterred.[66] By the middle of the sixteenth century, it was understood that damaging the brain could cause death, as it had with Henry II of France in 1559 when he had been killed by a lance piercing his eye and going into his brain. This medical understanding may explain why the Count had chosen to drive a nail through the head of this corpse to prevent it from rising again.

Manifestations of the vampire from the Middle Ages through the Enlightenment were not limited to a life in darkness, forced to return to the grave before being burned by the harsh rays of the sun. On the contrary, they were able to engage more fully with the living, with interactions as simple as a conversation or as complex as marrying and having children. Nighttime was, however, when the vampire needed to feed, often scouring the countryside looking for someone from whom to pull the essence of life. As vampires entered into the space of the living, their presence was used to explain things that were not easily understood.[67] Such interactions were considered in the origin story of the vampire, how corpses were reanimated, and what to do about it.

Regarding the origin story of the vampire in Europe, it was generally accepted that those who had been haunted by or fed on by vampires became vampires after they died, and the cycle repeated. This belief gave way to fear and concerns about the dead remaining dead. The reason that corpses reanimated was of particular concern. While the lack of understanding about human anatomy and physiology sometimes resulted in people being incorrectly diagnosed as dead, historic vampire accounts and reports of people being prematurely buried did not have the same characteristics. There are precious few stories of vampires with bloody hands or feet, cuts along their arms or legs, or broken noses, which were common in descriptions of confirmed premature burials. Conversely, narratives of premature diagnosis or burial also included characteristics such as someone thinking that they saw the body move, noises or screams coming from the grave, and an eventual exhumation with the intent to save the person's life. However, rather than calling to be freed from their graves, vampires were able to release themselves. Likewise, the bodies of vampires were not reported as being twisted or tortured when their grave was opened; instead they appeared to be resting and full of blood. Vampires were not believed to have been prematurely buried. It was believed that vampires reanimated due to the spirit waking up prior to the Reckoning.

In 1597, King James VI of Scotland (1566–1625) declared that devil possession was responsible for the reanimation of a corpse. In contrast to the majority of his Protestant subjects, he believed that the devil was able to enter into a dead body because the body was devoid of the soul and, therefore, vulnerable. The empty corpse was considered to be more vulnerable than a living person where the connection between the body and soul was expected to be strong enough to keep the devil away. There was not widespread belief in the devil's ability to raise a corpse. Rather, some people felt that the belief in vampires stemmed from superstitious nonsense or was "the product of deranged minds."[68] Even when the concept was considered practically, the idea of the devil entering a rotting corpse was considered to go against the natural order, a generally disgusting and fruitless proposition. According to a discourse on "Spirits and Divels" (1601), if the devil tried to reanimate a rotting corpse, the body would not be fit for use.[69] This dismissiveness helped establish the vampire's superstitious roots in folklore. The reanimated corpse was considered to be neither living nor dead. Rather it was thought to be something else entirely, a threshold person, and so had to be treated differently. Whether evil or confused, it was believed that the soul was so strong that it could take control of the body and force it out of the grave and back into the life that the person had previously lived. Another theory was that the recovered dead had been excommunicated, which was why they had been rejected by the earth after having been buried. In order to counter this rejection, those whose sanctity was deemed worthy or necessary were buried with a holy wafer in their mouth.

Once a vampire had risen from its grave, those it interacted with had a variety of ways that they could respond, based on what was already understood about the undead. As identified in the Count de Cabreras' report, certain medical values were understood. It was understood that the blood of a living person presented differently than that of a dead person. It was understood that since the loss of blood caused death, those who returned from the dead were hungry for blood. It was understood that damaging the brain could cause death. It was understood that the soul was considered to be the essence or spark of life. Armed with this medical knowledge, those who encountered a vampire were able to use this information to their advantage.

More often than not people were alarmed by the return of the deceased. The concepts of apparent and absolute death, as well as the signs of life and death were still being identified during the middle of the eighteenth century. This meant that people were often left with the fraught responsibility of making sure that whatever action was taken against the no-longer-dead person resulted in a permanent demise. One of the most popular ways of dealing with a vampiric corpse was to drive a pointed piece of metal, generally iron, through the vampire's torso. In some cases, substantial blood loss was reported. In others, the corpse awoke and screamed in agony before its ultimate demise. Another method included removing the head of the corpse and placing it separately from the body or removing it from the grave entirely. This was done in the case of the chieftain Abhartach, who also had a boulder placed over his grave to ensure that he could not rise from the ground. There were also reports of reaping tools, such as sickles, placed over the neck of a corpse. In traditional vampire folklore, sickles were supposed to ward away evil. Therefore, it was believed that securing one across the neck of a vampire would keep the being in place because it would not want its neck to touch the metal blade. Sometimes a brick or large stone was put into the mouth or around the throat of the corpse. This was intended to keep the vampire from chewing through its shroud, enabling it to get out of its grave. Additionally, sometimes the jaw was wrapped closed to keep a reanimated body from being able to chew through the burial shroud or winding sheet.

Reports of vampires chewing through their shrouds were especially prevalent in Germany. The word "nachzehrer" was used to describe corpses who reanimated in their graves and chewed on their shrouds. Modernly, we know that as the body decomposes, the lining of the gastrointestinal tract breaks down. This process causes dark red fluid to come out of the nose and the mouth. The intestines become bloated as gasses build up within the decomposing body. When the body enters rigor mortis, the mouth opens and the shroud could easily fall into it and stick to the blood, making it look as though the corpse is chewing on its shroud and had recently ingested blood. The noise generated by supposed chewing through the shroud was described as being so loud that it sounded like pigs at the trough to those above ground. In actuality, the sounds were likely heard while the corpses waited for burial. It was unlikely that the sound of the pressure changing and the bones and muscles shifting during decomposition could be heard through the earth once the body had been buried.

During the seventeenth and eighteenth centuries, there was a profound interest in vampire literature and lore. Medical, political, and religious facts blended with superstition, the supernatural, and outright fiction to create a whirlwind of vampire reports in books, letters, and literature. As the reported incidents mounted, people became concerned about the number of stories that were cropping up throughout Europe. Stories about vampire encounters in both Eastern and Western Europe were published and made available to the British audience. Newspaper reports helped spread the word of vampire experiences throughout Europe. Although many people believed that vampires were real and posed a threat to their health and life, not everyone held this opinion. The British newspaper the *Newcastle Courant* published information from a letter from Vienna, which was sent on June 21, 1738. The letter referenced other letters from Temeswaer, Romania in which the author explained that the "ridiculous Opinion of Vampires, which was so much talk'd of four of five Years ago, is again revived."[70] The author went on to define vampires as "dead Bodies [that] rise out of their Graves, and suck the Blood of People asleep; after which they believe that the Persons suck'd become, in their Turn, Vampires."[71] Like the stories published over the centuries before, those who were assumed to be vampires were beheaded and a stake was driven through their hearts. The author was of the mind that those who believed in vampires were ignorant and superstitious. However, like the story of Vesalius' premature dissection of a young Spanish noble, the questionable validity of vampire stories was historically important because people believed in them.

In 1786, the *Reading Mercury and Oxford Gazette* published a story that showcased how people could appear to be both alive and dead. A man had been walking along Clare Street in Bristol, England when he heard a woman shouting for help. He and a watchman, who also heard the woman shouting, attended the house where her cries seemed to emanate from.

Here they were conducted by a female into a small room; where a man lay stretched upon the floor and appeared to be dead; his features seemed to be quite fixed, and his face was besmeared with blood. On lifting his hand, it was observed to retain some warmth, but when let go it fell to the floor as if lifeless. By this time the room was crouded [*sic*] with females of the most wretched description and appearance, accompanied by a man who was asserted to be the murderer by the female who introduced the gentleman, and who in consequence was, with the assistance of the night constable and other watchmen that came in, taken into custody. But, now the seene [*sic*] materially changed; for the supposed murdered man suddenly started up, and on examining him was found not to have received the least injury. He had long since lost his right eye, but blood being smeared over the part, it appeared as if recently done. But the supposed murderer and murdered were immediately conveyed to Bridewell.[72]

John Polidori's (1795–1821) story *The Vampyre* had a similar narrative to the article published in the *Reading Mercury and Oxford Gazette*, where the main character was convinced that his companion had died until he saw him again. Polidori was a physician who had earned his medical degree at the University of Edinburgh in 1815 at the age of 19. During his medical training, he focused his research on sleepwalking. The following year, he was hired on as Lord Byron's personal physician. Polidori accompanied Byron as he toured through Europe and was with him in Geneva. While there, he became quite enthralled with the young Mary Godwin.

Polidori and Godwin discussed various medical topics including madness, vaccinations, and patient confidentiality. Over time, Polidori and Byron's relationship became estranged and eventually diminished. Conversely, Godwin viewed Polidori as her younger brother, despite the fact that he was actually older than her. During the especially rainy summer of 1816, Polidori, Byron, and Godwin discussed ghost stories that had been recently published. Byron read a few of the verses of Coleridge's *Christabel* and excerpts from the German anthology of ghost stories, *Phantasmagoria*. In this atmosphere, Byron issued the challenge that they should all try their hand at writing their own ghost stories. In response to this challenge, Mary (Godwin) Shelley wrote *Frankenstein* (1818), John Polidori wrote *The Vampyre* (1819), and Lord Byron wrote a short story titled *The Fragment of a Novel* (1819). Although *Frankenstein* is more of a cautionary tale of the responsibility of medical ethics, it still included a bit about vampirism. Shelley included this line as Victor recalled the death of his brother: "I considered the being whom I had cast among mankind, and endowed with the will and power to effect purposes of horror, such as the deed which he had now done, nearly in the light of my own vampire, my own spirit set loose from the grave, and forced to destroy all that was dear to me."[73]

The introduction of Polidori's *The Vampyre* included a history of the superstitions regarding vampires. Polidori repeated the story of Arnold Paul before going on to explain that, in Greece, vampirism was considered to be a type of punishment that took place after death. People were sometimes condemned to this postmortem punishment if they had committed a "heinous crime" during their lifetime.[74] He also gave credence to vampire stories that had come before, listing parts of *A Fragment of a Turkish Tale* and *Thalaba the Destroyer* as evidence that literary vampires came back to life in order torment those that they had once loved or felt a kinship to. Finally, he included historical research on vampires that had been published during the eighteenth century, such as the information published by Calmet.

The Vampyre is a story of seduction and the living dead. It introduced the handsome, well dressed, aristocratic vampire into the genre. Similar in personality to Coleridge's female seductress, Polidori's vampire was a male who seduced aristocratic women, enchanting them before sucking out their blood. It has been generally accepted that the main character, the vampire, Lord Ruthven was modeled after Lord Byron. Therefore, it should not come as a surprise that Polidori modeled Lord Ruthven's traveling companion, Aubrey, after himself. During the first half of the story, Aubrey often enjoyed the company of a young woman, Ianthe, whom he considered to be so ethereal that she was practically a fairy. During one of their many talks, she imparted to him "the tale of the living vampire, who had passed years amidst his friends, and dearest ties, forced every year, by feeding upon the life of a lovely female to prolong his existence for the ensuing months."[75] Although Aubrey did not want to believe her story, Ianthe shared the names of people who knew that vampires were living among them. She explained that they had markings indicating that they had been recently fed upon.

Later in the story, Ianthe died and when Aubrey was shown her "lifeless corpse," it was noted that she had "no colour upon her cheek, not even upon her lip; yet there was a stillness about her face that seemed almost as attaching as the life that once dwelt there:—upon her neck and breast was blood, and upon her throat were the marks of teeth having opened the vein."[76] Upon seeing her colorless corpse and the bite marks upon her neck, the people who brought her body to Aubrey identified that these were the signs that she had been attacked by a vampire. Soon thereafter, Aubrey identified Lord Ruthven as the vampire. Even as his trust for his companion waned, Lord Ruthven took care of him as he recovered from the shock of losing Ianthe.

Lord Ruthven and Aubrey decided to travel through parts of Greece that they had not seen before. While on their journey, they were accosted by robbers and Lord Ruthven was shot in the shoulder. As the days passed by, his body weakened, although he looked and acted the same as he ever had. Soon thereafter Lord Ruthven appeared to have died, and Aubrey was informed that the body had been laid out upon a rock. Intent on ensuring that Lord Ruthven remained dead, Aubrey went to bury him. When he was unable to locate the body, he assumed that it had already been buried, and he decided to return home to England. Upon his return home, he began to see Lord Ruthven in crowded spaces and in his dreams. Soon after, Aubrey fell ill and was unable to get out of bed for days at a time. As the months drifted by, his health continued to decline, and he began to take on the appearance of death.

During his illness, he learned that his sister had become engaged to an Earl—who turned out to be Lord Ruthven. Since Aubrey had failed to confirm his death in Greece, and it gave Ruthven time to recover from his wound and return to London. Aubrey's illness had kept him out of the way, which allowed Lord Ruthven the time to court his sister. Due to Aubrey's diminishing health, he was not able to prevent the marriage. By the time he was able to request that his sister visit, it was too late. His sister had been "glutted" to quench the thirst of the vampire, and Lord Ruthven had disappeared.[77]

When the story is compared to a historical vampire story, there are some interesting twists in the narrative. Lord Ruthven had already been identified as the vampire, and his initial death and reanimation were not discussed in the story. Throughout *The Vampyre*, Polidori mentioned the signs and symptoms of death. When writing about Ianthe's corpse, he noted the stillness of her corpse and that the color had drained from her face. When describing Aubrey's illness, he mentioned that his eyes became glassy and he lost a considerable amount of weight. Polidori's training as a physician allowed him to be cognizant of the signs of death. Therefore, his statement that Lord Ruthven looked and acted the same even as he appeared to die was purposeful foreshadowing that he was not actually dying. The foreshadowing was echoed when Ruthven's body disappeared when it was laid out for viewing but could not be found for burial. Therefore, it cannot be said that he returned from the grave, because he had not been put into one. Ruthven did return home—albeit Aubrey's home—and interacted with the living. The story was rife with the implication that Lord Ruthven was drinking the blood of the living, which was how Aubrey knew that his sister was in danger. In these ways, Polidori took the signs that had historically been attributed to the vampire and reassigned them to different aspects of his story.

An analysis of vampire literature would not be complete without touching upon Bram Stoker's *Dracula*. Of the man Bram Stoker (1847–1912), some things are known and some things have been assumed. He did not leave many personal writings for future scholars to study. Therefore, much of the information that has been collected about him has been derived from correspondence, notes, and business paperwork. It is known that he was born in Ireland in 1847 and that he was sickly as a child. When he was of age, he attended Trinity College (Dublin) to study mathematics. He never traveled to Eastern Europe, so most of his descriptions were derived from secondary accounts. It is known that he became the Victorian actor Sir Henry Irving's business manager. It has been assumed that he was either gay or bisexual. Just as information about Stoker's life were implied through social cues in his limited documentary papers, social connections to sexuality and vampirism were hidden within the text of his book *Dracula*.

In the past several decades scholars have noticed the emphasis that Stoker put on sexuality. This was particularly noticeable in the female characters, who were both "wildly erotic, and motivated by an insatiable thirst for blood."[78] In this way they are a combination of the Coleridge's femme fatale vampire from *Christabel*, the female vampire who continues to show the signs of life and have a thirst for blood from Sheridan's *Carmilla*, and the popular culture favorite aristocratic blood sucking fiend from Polidori's *The Vampyre*. The epitome of Gothic horror fiction, this masterpiece has been read, and subsequently analyzed, for over a century. Regarded as a classic, this story makes certain that the reader never forgets their journey through early modern medicine, if they know where to look.

Like *The Vampyre*, the entire tale of *Dracula* is one of vampirism. Unlike most vampires, it is alluded that Dracula had taught himself how to turn into a vampire by studying so many subjects that his "brain powers survived the physical death."[79] This idea emphasized the understanding that the brain must keep working in order for the body to survive and implied that as long as the brain continued to function, the body could become immortal. After one of the main protagonists of the novel, Jonathan Harker, realized that he had been taken prisoner by Count Dracula, he decided to explore the castle. Finding himself in a small chapel, he walked down into the vaults. While exploring there, he noticed fragments of coffins in two of the vaults and found Count Dracula entranced in the third vault, laying in a box "on a pile of newly dug earth."[80] As he looked on, Harker realized that he could not tell if the Count was alive or dead. This confusion was due to the mixed signals that he observed regarding the conflicting signs of life and death. Harker recalled that the Count could have been alive because his open eyes did not hold the glassy look of death. Likewise, his cheeks "had the warmth of life through all their pallor," and his lips were red.[81] However, Harker could not detect any sign of breathing or a pulse.

The next time that Harker went to the Count's vault, he opened the coffin and noticed that the Count seemed to be younger; his gray hair had become darker, and his face was fatter. A curious addition to his countenance was blood on his lips. Harker described the Count as looking like he was "simply gorged with blood."[82] In this description, it appeared as though Stoker pulled from the descriptions of vampire burials which had been recorded in the preceding century. This theory is further supported by Harker's next action. Grabbing a shovel, he raised it up and began to stab the Count in the face. Harker became startled when the Count's head turned towards him, and he missed when he brought the shovel back down, hitting the Count in the forehead instead. Since the shovel was ostensibly metal, this echoes the superstition that a vampire corpse needed to be impaled with a metal object, either through the chest or by cutting off its head. Having been unable to complete either action, Harker accidentally allowed the Count to live, and as a result, he wreaks havoc upon several other characters throughout the book. However, Dracula is not the character that best exemplifies a historically accurate vampire encounter in this book.

Back in England, Harker's fiancée, Mina, was visiting her friend, Lucy, at the coastal town of Whitby. One night, Mina realized that Lucy had left their room and she followed her to the town's cemetery. There Mina noticed a tall, lanky figure leaning over her seated friend. After chasing off the shadowy figure, Mina clasped a cloak around her friend's shoulders and brought her back to their room. Upon removing the cloak, she noticed two little pin pricks on Lucy's throat and a drop of blood on the collar of her nightgown. She becomes concerned that she had clasped the safety pin through her friend's neck, but Lucy insisted that she did not feel the injury. After Lucy's encounter in the cemetery, she began to have trouble breathing and became increasingly weak for a prolonged period of time. Months later, when the wounds were observed by Dr. John Seward, and his mentor, Professor Van Helsing, it was noticed that they had not healed, and they wondered if the marks on her neck were the cause of her prolonged illness.

It was determined that her body was weakened by a great loss of blood and that she would die without a blood transfusion. After a partial blood transfusion, from her fiancé Arthur, Lucy's coloring brightens. After Stoker made use of Polidori's concept of a vampire leaving bite marks on the victim's neck, he also identified the need for blood to sustain life. However, rather than having Lucy drink the blood that she so craved, he relied on medical advances that had been made during the nineteenth century and gave her a blood transfusion. Despite the transfusion, Lucy died.

During Lucy's funeral, she showed the symptoms of both life and death. She was not breathing, and her heart did not beat. But her body was not decaying, and her face was still described as "beautiful." During her wake, Van Helsing placed wild garlic around her bed and put his crucifix upon her lips. He also wanted to remove her heart and her head from her body. By the late nineteenth century these were well known ways of ensuring that vampires did not return. Unfortunately, the crucifix was removed before her burial, which caused Van Helsing to be skeptical that she would stay within her coffin. To validate his skepticism, he and Seward opened her coffin and found it empty, just as he had anticipated. While Van Helsing believed that this proved that she was a vampire, Seward believed that her body had been stolen by a resurrectionist or the coroner. It was not until the next night when they returned to Lucy's grave and reopened her coffin that Seward began to believe that something might be amiss. Lucy now lay within her coffin, even "more radiantly beautiful" than she had looked during her wake the week before.[83] Her lips were bright red, and her cheeks were pink. Her canine teeth had become sharper, and she had not decayed in the slightest. Van Helsing believed that the best course of action was to place garlic in her mouth and kill her by beheading her and driving a stake through her torso.

Instead, they shared Lucy's plight with Arthur. As they explained the situation and that Lucy might not be entirely dead, Arthur asked if there had been a mistake which caused her to be buried alive. Like the possibility of the corpse being stolen, this was a much more logical conclusion than the theory that Lucy had been turned into a vampire. The men returned once more to her coffin. Upon opening the lid, they found the coffin empty like it had been on the first night. They later encountered the undead Lucy when she returned from her hunt for blood. She is alluring, cruel, and has blood dripping from her lips and onto her burial garments. Seward described the sight as a "Thing" which has "taken Lucy's shape without her soul."[84] They returned the next day and Van Helsing explained that according to vampire lore, the undead were unable to die and, instead, "must go on age after age adding new victims and multiplying the evils of the world; for all that die from the preying of the Un-Dead becomes themselves Un-Dead, and prey on their kind.... But if she die in truth, then all cease; the tiny wounds of the throats disappear, and they [the children she hunted] go back to their plays unknowing ever of what has been."[85] After learning this, Arthur hammers a stake into Lucy's heart, effectively killing her and allowing the body to finally rest in peace.

Of the different vampire stories within Stoker's *Dracula*, Lucy's most resembled that of a historical vampire. The reanimation of her corpse was exemplified by the way that she disappeared and reappeared within her coffin. Likewise, the proof that she *left* her "final" resting place, rather than her body being taken by resurrectionists, was indicated by the confrontation between herself and the group of men who set out to destroy her. Although Lucy did not return to the home that she shared with her fiancé, Arthur, she did return to the town. Once there, she drank the blood of those weaker than herself, namely children. After she had her fill, she returned back to her grave. By completing all of these actions, Lucy's story in *Dracula* fulfilled the five concepts of a historical vampire story.

The creation of the vampire in popular culture has been derived from centuries of vampire lore culminated with vampire fiction. The literary vampire has taken many forms, from the femme fatale to a supernatural being to the alluring aristocrat. Whether the character was of humble upbringings or noble birth, they all had a strong survival instinct. Whether through deceit or direct engagement, they all stalked their prey and drew the life force out of the living, taking it for their own. Writers included medical theory as it was known to them. Even as the medical theory changed, the core characteristics of the vampire story remained the same, rooted strongly in the history of medicine.

Conclusion

"The custom of hastily laying out the persons supposed to be dead, and rashly interring the same, has been opposed, by men of learning and philanthropy, in this and other countries."[1]

Initial analyses of current scholarly material relating to the evolution of thought on burial customs, medical theory, and the sale of the corpse, have shown a call and response pattern between society and the medical community. The call and response cycle between the public and the medical community had been long standing. When people were being misdiagnosed as dead during ancient times, the scholars of the era wrote about the situation and presented a plea to future scholars to fix the issue since they could not. When people continued to be misdiagnosed as dead through the Renaissance, the story of Vesalius' mistake in prematurely dissecting a young noble became so widespread that it fell into popular history and was repeated for centuries as an example of how even the best could misdiagnose someone as dead.

As society became aware that people were being misdiagnosed as dead and the premature repercussions that occurred as a result, the public turned to the medical community for answers. In turn, the medical community acknowledged that people were being misdiagnosed as dead, which resulted in the evolution of how the definition, stages, and signs of death were understood. Concurrently, there was a shortage of cadavers for anatomical dissections, so the medical community relied on resurrectionists to obtain the numbers of cadavers necessary. The acceptance of the sale of corpses culminated in two sets of resurrectionist gangs (one in England, one in Scotland) who turned to murder to fulfill the requests during the 1820s and 1830s. When the public became aware of these murders, it broke the trust between society and the medical community. Although this research focuses on the implications of misdiagnosed death and how the medical community and society at large responded, the resurrectionist's involvement is an important part of both narratives. The

172

consequences of these murders brought this era of British medicine to a close with the Anatomy Act of 1832.

It has been generally accepted that the misdiagnosis of death caused people to be prematurely buried during the eighteenth century. The relationship between the public's awareness of the issue and the medical community's response to further identify the signs and symptoms of death has not been previously explored. While researching reported cases of misdiagnosed death, there were four bodily outcomes. People were (1) either enclosed in their coffins, (2) buried in their grave, (3) interred in their tomb, or (4) the body was repurposed for anatomical dissection. Textual evidence of these outcomes exists in the form of state papers, Parliamentary reports, newspapers, books, pamphlets, and literature. By creating the term "premature repercussions," I was able to condense these outcomes into one cohesive concept. The action of resuscitation was not included with the premature repercussions because it was a process acted upon the body for the expressed purpose of rousing the individual. Conversely, the watching of the body, burial/interment, and possible disinterment of the body for dissection were regular parts of the burial process.

It was serendipity that the interest in properly identifying the signs of death was renewed during the middle of the eighteenth century, just as medical theory had advanced to the point where answers could be discovered. Previously accepted medical advancements, such as dissecting humans to study human anatomy and physiology and the acceptance of William Tossach's resuscitative method formed the foundation of the medical community's ability to respond. Despite many advances in medicine, people continued to be diagnosed as apparently dead because deeper knowledge regarding anatomy and physiology was only starting to evolve out of a basic understanding. As of 1771, the definition of death was still as simple as the body not being alive and having separated from the soul. Although the latter was eminently difficult to prove, the former was in the process of detection and understanding throughout the eighteenth century. Physicians such as Drs. John Fothergill, Alexander Johnson, Charles Kite, James Curry, and Anthony Fothergill worked to develop a more comprehensive definition of death, and that definition progressed alongside the evolving understanding of human anatomy and physiology. The most common signs of death that they identified were the cessation of automatic functions, the cessation of respiration and a heartbeat, and the departure of the soul from the body.

The evolution of the definition of death during the eighteenth century has been a largely unexplored element of the history of medicine. The research being done to explain how human anatomy and physiology were affected by the process of dying had not yet been confirmed or broadly accepted. This caused people to be prematurely diagnosed as dead, and some of them suffered premature repercussions as a result. In 1744, William Tossach published a new method—the resuscitative process—used to revive people who were presenting as apparently dead due to suffocation. This method was revolutionary because it could be used on everyone who had been prematurely diagnosed as dead and could prevent them from suffering from premature repercussions. In 1745, Dr. John Fothergill published his approval of the resuscitative process in *Observations on the Recovery of a Man Dead in Appearance by Distending the Lungs with Air.* The following year, Jean-Benigne Winslow published *The Uncertainty of the Signs of Death and the Danger of Precipitate Interment* (1746), which focused on the prevalence of premature burial throughout European history. As these publications released, there was an increased interest in the study of medicine, anatomy, and physiology in London. Medical professionals and students were required to procure their own cadavers in order to further their anatomical studies. Unfortunately, the number of bodies which could be legally obtained were far dwarfed by the number of bodies that were needed. Therefore, medical professionals turned to resurrectionists, who exhumed freshly buried bodies, in order to fill in the gap.

The medical community responded to the awareness of people being misdiagnosed as dead by accepting the resuscitative process and founding the Royal Humane Society in London. The members of the Society continued to research the best practices and methods to apply the resuscitative process and published them for use by the general public. Anyone who even attempted to use the resuscitative process was rewarded by the Society. By the 1760s, the resuscitative process had become so popular that chapters were being opened throughout Western Europe to enhance its usage. It became a widely accepted test for death, which also had the benefit of being able to revive the patient.

Even as the medical community advanced its understanding of anatomy and physiology to answer questions about life and death, the British public remained aware that those who were diagnosed as dead could still be alive. While some people contended that concerns of premature burial were alarmist, others cited the importance of traditions such as watching the dead for signs of life during the wake to validate their concerns. Likewise, coffins were created that would alert those on the outside if the person on the inside had been prematurely enclosed or buried, and were trying to escape. That such mechanisms were invented and produced speaks to the deep concerns held by at least a segment of the society.

All the while, medical practitioners continued to research, study, and dissect in order to figure out how the anatomy and physiology of the body worked. In order to obtain the number of cadavers needed, they were reliant on resurrectionists to disinter recently buried bodies for them.

Problems arose from two different directions. First, were the religious beliefs to consider. People feared that disinterring and dissecting a corpse would make it impossible for the body to rise at the time of the Reckoning. People feared for their immortal lives. Additionally, some resurrectionists resorted to murdering people in order to supply the medical community with the freshest bodies on the market. Over time the laws began to change to protect the poor from those who would try to profit of their dead bodies. Secondly, the general public were concerned about identifying those who had been incorrectly diagnosed as dead. In response, they took particular precautions to watch the dead body during the wake and continued to understand that the only true sign for death was putrefaction. Some people requested more drastic measures be taken after their own deaths and requested that their throats be slit prior to their burial, thus ensuring that they were not accidentally prematurely buried.

Reports of people having been misdiagnosed as dead and buried alive have been recorded throughout history. If a person was buried only in a shroud and the body was buried in a shallow grave or towards the top of a mass grave, it is plausible that the person could have crawled their way to freedom and then returned home. It is likely that they would still be weak from lack of food and water, could be suffering from mild oxygen deprivation, and were feasibly unhappy that they had been literally left for dead. Beginning in the Middle Ages in Europe, stories were recorded about people returning from the dead and threatening their loved ones once they returned home. In these cases, people were reported as being angry, lethargic, and hungry. They knocked on the door, windows, walls, and roofs, trying to gain entrance to the home. Some were reported as resuming their place at the dinner table, hungry for their next meal. If they had been in an apparently dead state due to an illness, their return could have infected their family, inadvertently causing their deaths. An actual return from the grave many months or years after a person had been buried is more difficult to explain away; historically, such people have been called vampires.

When observers noticed that the body had not decayed as expected, causes for this seemingly atypical behavior were explored. Rigor mortis was added as a sign of death in the late nineteenth century. When a body goes into rigor mortis, the muscles and joints become stiff. This process generally begins a few hours after death and can continue for several days. Afterwards, the body becomes soft and pliable again. The return of this pliancy was sometimes misunderstood as a possible sign of life. Signs of decay might be overlooked in consequence. People of the eighteenth century and before were waiting for the body to rot outright. Much like the lack of information regarding the process of death, there was also a lack of information regarding the process of a decaying body. Both death and putrefaction became medicalized in the late nineteenth century. Therefore, stories such as Joan Bridges, Laurence Cawthorn, and Arnold Paul were all observed, perceived, and recorded without advanced medical understanding.

Fears of the dead returning were shared by the dying and those that they might return to. Threatening behavior of the no-longer-buried could take the form of physical violence or by bringing about disease, most often the plague. While it is easy to consider these to be extremist tales and flights of fancy, people did believe that vampires had returned from the dead. This is evidenced by several apparent vampire burials that were located in the late twentieth and early twenty-first centuries. These graves included decapitated or disjointed corpses to keep the body from being able to reanimate, stones or bricks shoved into the mouth to keep the person from being able to chew through their shroud, the destruction of the heart, and metal stakes being driven through their chest which destroyed the lungs and secured the corpse to the ground. Not only did these actions show that people were afraid that bodies were going to reanimate, but they also indicated an understanding that the brain, heart, and lungs were necessary to sustain life. It was already understood that these three organs were the nucleus of human life, even if it was not yet understood why.

Edgar Allan Poe once said, "To be buried while alive is, beyond question, the most terrific of these extremes which has ever fallen to the lot of mere mortality."[2] Premature burial ... coming back from the dead ... people returning home after their own funeral. These sound like plot lines for B-rated horror stories, the likes of which were spoofed by *Mystery Science Theater 3000*. The concept of people still being alive after being buried in the grave, or enclosed (while living) into their final resting places has inspired horror authors for generations. But this macabre topic did not originate in the darkest recesses of the minds of fanciful authors. Instead, it was a real predicament that befell people while the medical community attempted to identify what precisely constituted death.

Early hypotheses regarding the prevalence of premature burial were reported in British sources in 1793 and 1817. In 1793, it was hypothesized that between 10 percent and 50 percent of those who were diagnosed as dead and then buried throughout Western Europe were still alive. In 1817, it was hypothesized that 10 percent of English people who were diagnosed as dead and subsequently buried were still alive. Two hundred (200) cases of apparent death, which had occurred in Europe and places of British extension (America, India, or a military ship/outpost) and were reported by British sources, were collected and analyzed for this book. An analysis of the collected cases indicated that 29 individuals, or 14.5 percent of the total cases of apparent death resulted in a premature repercussion, and that 55 percent of the 29 individuals were prematurely buried or interred. Further analysis of those 29 cases suggested a survival rate of 65.5 percent. More narrowly assessed, of the 130 cases that occurred in England or a place of British extension, seven individuals (5.4 percent) incurred in a premature repercussion. These seven cases had nearly a 99 percent survival rate. When compared to the hypothesized rate of misdiagnosed death from 1793 and 1817, the assertions made by Baron de Hupch and John Snart best align with the results of this study.

This new information on the prevalence of misdiagnosed death and premature repercussions that victims suffered during the eighteenth century opens new avenues of study relating to social, economic, and medical history in England and Europe. Future scholars will also have the ability to expand and compare the number of cases of apparent death and the consequences experienced during later eras and other locales. For example, the relevance of this research is similar to the ongoing research being done by the Museum of London Archeology (MOLA). In 2018, the MOLA began working with HS2 to exhume the St. James Garden Cemetery in order to create a new Underground line. This project has approved the exhumation of the roughly 61,000 bodies that were buried in St. James Gardens between 1790 and 1853, with the intent to rebury them elsewhere. If, for example, the demographic information that was analyzed in my study was coupled with osteoarchaeological information made accessible during this mass exhumation, the larger sample size would allow for a more accurate modern representation of the number of misdiagnosed deaths and premature burials. Although winding sheets and wooden coffins are likely to have already disintegrated, lead or iron coffins may have remained intact. Additionally, in cases where the structure of the skeleton remained relatively in place, observation of the bones would indicate if they were in the expected position or if they appeared to have moved after burial. Anthropological assessments could indicate if any bone breaks or stress fractures occurred on the forearms, forehead, knees, feet, shins, or hands, and how much they had healed prior to the person's death. Similarly, (depending how airtight the coffin was) the insides of coffins could be analyzed to see if there are any indentations, scratch marks, or dried blood remaining, which would indicate that its inhabitant had tried to escape. If the percentages reported in my initial case study remained objectively similar to the St. James Cemetery dig, this would increase the number of misdiagnosed deaths in England from 130 to over 39,500 people and the number of premature burials from three to over 900—just from this one cemetery. This would prove that even if only a small percentage of the larger number of people were being misdiagnosed as dead and prematurely buried, it still impacted many people. This would help clarify why so many people were afraid of being misdiagnosed as dead even as others considered the concept to be alarmist.

Appendix: Source List for Cases of Apparent Death Misdiagnosed as Death

The 200 cases that were misdiagnosed as death and were analyzed for premature repercussions came from primary and secondary books and newspapers published during or soon after the period of investigation. The primary and secondary books were chosen because they were written by medical practitioners who were respected in their fields. The newspapers were located by searching through the following collections: British Newspaper Archive (British Library), the National Archives (England), 17th–18th Century Burney Collection (Gale Group), and 17th and 18th Century Nichols Newspaper Collection (Farmington Hills Gale/Cengage Learning). The pamphlets were located in the Eighteenth Century Collections Online (Gale/Cengage Learning). The newspaper and pamphlets were located via keyword search and chosen to be used because they included relevant information with enough demographic information to appear valid. The materials gathered represent an exhaustive search of the available literature—the only cases that were exempted from analysis were those with incomplete data and those with questionable authenticity.

While some of the sources were searchable in an online format, others were accessed by visiting the British Library, the Royal College of Physicians, and the London Metropolitan Archive. Key points of each case were screened by the author, Nicole Salomone, to determine accuracy and authenticity. Complete citations for the books and pamphlets are located in the bibliography.

Primary Sources

Books

Buchan, William. *Domestic Medicine; Or, a Treatise on the Prevention and Cure of Diseases by Regimen and Simple Medicines. With an Appendix,*

Containing a Dispensatory for the Use of Private Practitioners. London: A. Strahan; T. Cadell, 1791.

Curry, James. *Observations on Apparent Death from Drowning, Suffocation, &c. With an Account of the Means to be Employed for Recovery: Drawn up at the Desire of the Northamptonshire Preservative Society.* Northampton: Dicey and Co., 1792.

Hawes, William. *An Address to the King and Parliament of Great Britain on Preserving the Lives of the Inhabitants.* London: J. Dodsely, 1783.

Hawes, William. *An Address to the Public.* London: H. Goldney, 1779.

Hawes, William. *Royal Humane Society ... Annual Report.* London: J. Nichols, 1798.

Hawes, William. *Royal Humane Society ... Annual Report.* London: J. Nicholas, 1799.

Jackson, Rowland. *A Physical Dissertation on Drowning.* London: Jacob Robinson, 1746.

Johnson, Alexander. *A Collection of Authentic Cases Proving the Practicability of Recovering Personal Visibly Dead by Drowning, Suffocation, Stifling, Swooning, Convulsions, and Other Accidents.* London: John Nourse, 1775.

Smythson, Hugh. *The Compleate Family Physician, Or Universal Medical Repository.* London: Harrison and Co., 1785.

Struve, Christian. *A Practical Essay on the Art of Recovering Suspended Animation.* London: Murray and Highley, 1802.

Taylor, Joseph. *The Danger of Premature Interment Proved from Many Remarkable Instances of People Who Have Recovered After Being Laid Out for Dead.* London: W. Simpkin and R. Marshall, 1816.

Winslow, Jean-Benigne. *The Uncertainty of the Signs of Death and the Danger of Precipitate Interments and Dissections.* London: The Globe, 1746.

Newspapers

Aberdeen Press and Journal (Aberdeen, Aberdeenshire, Scotland)

Argus (London, London, England)

Bath Chronicle and Weekly Gazette (Bath, Somerset, England)

Bury and Norwich Post (Bury St. Edmunds, Suffolk, England)

Caledonian Mercury (Edinburgh, Midlothian, Scotland)

Chelmsford Chronicle (Chelmsford, Essex, England)

Chester Chronicle (Chester, Cheshire, England)

Chester Courant (Chester, Cheshire, England)

The Courier (Dundee, Dundee, Scotland)

Cumberland Pacquet and Ware's Whitehaven Advertiser (Whitehaven, Cumberland, England)

Derby Mercury (Derby, Derbyshire, England)

Evening Mail (London, London, England)

Felix Farley's Bristol Journal (Bristol, Bristol, England)
Gazetteer and New Daily Advertiser (London, London, England)
General Evening Post (London, London, England)
Gloucester Journal (Gloucester, Gloucestershire, England)
Hampshire Chronicle (Winchester, Hampshire, England)
Hereford Journal (Hereford, Herefordshire, England)
Hibernian Journal; or, Chronicle of Liberty (Dublin, Dublin, Republic of
    Ireland)
The Ipswich Journal (Ipswich, Suffolk, England)
Kentish Gazette (Canterbury, Kent, England)
Leeds Intelligencer (Leeds, Yorkshire, England)
The London Chronicle (London, London, England)
Middlesex Journal (London, London, England)
Morning Chronicle (London, London, England)
Newcastle Courant (Newcastle-upon-Tyne, Northumberland, England)
Norfolk Chronicle (Norwich, Norfolk, England)
Northampton Mercury (Northampton, Northamptonshire, England)
The Oracle (London, London, England)
Oxford Journal (Oxford, Oxfordshire, England)
Public Advertiser (London, London, England)
Reading Mercury (Reading, Berkshire, England)
Reading Mercury and Oxford Gazette (Reading, Berkshire, England)
St. James's Chronicle or the British Evening Post (London, London, England)
Salisbury and Winchester Journal (Salisbury, Wiltshire, England)
Saunder's News-Letter (Dublin, Dublin, Republic of Ireland)
The Scots Magazine (Edinburgh, Midlothian, Scotland)
Staffordshire Advertiser (Stafford, Staffordshire, England)
Stamford Mercury (Stamford, Lincolnshire, England)
Star and Evening Advertiser (London, London, England)
The Times (London, London, England)
The True Briton (London, London, England)
White Evening Post (London, London, England)
Whitehall Evening Post (London, London, England)

Pamphlets

Anonymous. *A Brief history of John Bubble and Thomas Greenman.* Dublin,
    1735.
Anonymous. *A new prophesy: Or, An Account of a young Girl, not above Eight
    Years of Age Who being in a trance, or lay as dead for the Space of 48 Hours.*
    London?, 1780.
Anonymous. *The Surprising Wonder of Doctor Watts, Who Lay in a Trance
    Three Days. To Which Is Added, a Sermon, Preached at His Intended Funeral.*
    London?, 1710.

Secondary Sources

Books

Bailey, James Blake. *Diary of a Resurrectionist (1811–1812)*. London: Swan Sonnanschein & Co., 1896.

Tebb, William. *Premature Burial and How It May Be Prevented*. London: Swan Sonnanschein & Co., 1905.

Tebb, William, and Vollum, Col. Edward Perry. *Premature Burial and How It May Be Prevented*. London: Swan Sonnenschien & Co., 1896.

Chapter Notes

Introduction

1. "Wonderful Escape of a Sailor from Being Buried Alive." *Times*, 16 Oct. 1788, p.4. *The Times Digital Archive*, http://tinyurl.galegroup.com/tinyurl/9BGTP4. Gale Document Number: GALE|CS6737 2880.

2. *Master and Commander*, directed by Peter Weir (2003; Los Angeles: Twentieth Century Fox), DVD.

Chapter 1

1. Joseph Taylor, *The Danger of Premature Interment, Proved from Many Remarkable Instances of People Who Have Recovered After Being Laid Out for Dead, ad of Others Entombed Alive, for Want of Being Properly Examined Prior to Interment* (London: W. Simpkin and R. Marshall, 1816), 25.

2. Taylor, *Danger of Premature Interment*, 26.

3. Taylor, *Danger of Premature Interment*, 26.

4. Jean-Benigne Winslow, *The Uncertainty of the Signs of Death and the Danger of Precipitate Interments and Dissections* (London: The Globe, 1746), 38.

5. Edited by the Wernerian Club, *Pliny's Natural History in Thirty-Seven Books. A Translation on the Basis of That by Dr. Philemon Holland, Ed. 1601. With Critical and Explanatory Notes* (London: George Barclay, 1847–48), Book VII, 241.

6. Wernerian Club, *Pliny's Natural History*, 242.

7. Wernerian Club, *Pliny's Natural History*, 243.

8. Aulus Cornelius Celsus, *A Literal Interlineal Translation of the First Four Books of Celsus De Medicina: With "Ordo" And Text: Tr. From the Text Selected for the Examination of Candidates at Apothecaries' Hall, And Other Public Boards; In Which the Elliptical Constructions Are Completed by Supplying the Suppressed Words, Shewing the Relations and Concords of the Different Words with Each Other*, 2d ed., translated by Robert Venables (London: Sherwood, Gilbert, and Piper, 1837), 71.

9. Lucius Apuleius, *Apologia and Florida of Apuleius of Madaura*, translated by H.E. Butler (Oxford: Clarendon Press, 1909; Kindle: Good Press, 2019).

10. Apuleius, *Apologia and Florida*.

11. Apuleius, *Apologia and Florida*.

12. Celsus, *A Literal Interlineal Translation*, 71.

13. Dorian Giesler Greenbaum, "Astronomy, Astrology, and Medicine," *Handbook of Archeoastronomy and Ethnoastronomy* (2014), 117–132, https://doi.org/10.1007/978-1-4614-6141-8_19.

14. Plato, *Selected Dialogues of Plato: The Benjamin Jowett Translation, Revised and with an Introduction by Hayden Pelliccia* (New York: The Modern Library, 2001), 182.

15. Arnold M. Katz and Phillis B. Katz, "Diseases of the Heart in the Works of Hippocrates," *British Cardiovascular Society: Heart* 24 (1962): 257.

16. Hippocrates, "On Ancient Medicine," MIT: The Internet Classics Archive, Part 5. Translated by Francis Adams, accessed December 11, 2017, http://classics.mit.edu/Hippocrates/ancimed.html.

17. Hippocrates, *On Ancient Medicine*, Part 5.

18. W.N. Mann, *Hippocratic Writings,* translated by J. Chadwick (Harmondsworth: Penguin,1983), 262.

19. Vivian Nutton, "The Seeds of Disease: An Explanation of Contagion and Infection from the Greeks to the Renaissance," *Medicine History* 27 (1983): 3.

20. J.C. Dalton, *Galen and Hippocrates* (New York: D. Appleton, 1873), 9.

21. Dalton, *Galen and Hippocrates,* 9.

22. Stanley G. Schultz, "William Harvey and the Circulation of the Blood: The Birth of a Scientific Revolution and Modern Physiology," *News in Physiological Sciences* 17, no. 5 (2002): 176, https://doi.org/10.1152/nips.01391.2002.

23. Dalton, *Galen and Hippocrates,* 6.

24. Joseph F. Borzelleca, "Paracelsus: Herald of Modern Toxicology," *Toxicological Sciences* 53, no. 1 (2000): 1.

25. Walter Pagel, *Paracelsus: An Introduction to Philosophical Medicine in the Era of the Renaissance* (London: S. Karger, 1982), 129.

26. Pagel, *Paracelsus,* 200.

27. Edited by Holmes Boynton, *The Beginnings of Modern Science: Scientific Writings of the 16th, 17th, and 18th Centuries* (Roslyn: Walter J. Black, Inc., 1948), 532.

28. Boynton, *The Beginnings of Modern Science,* 531.

29. Boynton, *The Beginnings of Modern Science,* 532.

30. F.P. Wilson, *The Plague in Shakespeare's London* (Oxford: Oxford University Press, 1927), 15.

31. Harold J. Cook, *The Decline of the Old Medical Regime in Stuart London* (Ithaca: Cornell University Press, 1986), 71.

32. Royal College of Physicians, "History of the Royal College of Physicians," Royal College of Physicians, accessed April 21, 2021. https://www.rcplondon.ac.uk/about-us/who-we-are/history-royal-college-physicians.

33. W.S.C. Copeman, "The Evolution of Anatomy and Surgery Under the Tudors," *Thomas Vicary Lecture Delivered at the Royal College of Surgeons of England* (1962): 7.

34. Ankur Aggarwal, "The Evolving Relationship Between Surgery and Medicine," *American Medical Association Journal of Ethics* 12, no. 2 (2010): 120, doi: 10.1001/virtualmentor.2010.12.2.mhst1-1002.

35. Copeman, "The Evolution of Anatomy and Surgery Under the Tudors," 7.

36. "An Act Concerning Barbers and Surgeons to Be of One Company," 1540, 32, Henry VIII, c. 42, 43. Parliamentary Archives.

37. "An Act Concerning Barbers and Surgeons to Be of One Company," 32, Henry VIII, c. 42, 43.

38. Royal College of Physicians, "Dead Bodies: Petition of R.C.P to the House of Commons for Bill to Make Prevision for Redress in Matter of College Obtaining Executed Bodies for Dissection," 18th c?. Envelope 55, p. 68. Cat of Legal Docs, 1, Royal College of Physicians, London.

39. Julia Bess Frank, "Body Snatching: A Grave Medical Problem," *The Yale Journal of Biology and Medicine* 49 (1976): 400.

40. Paul W. Glimcher, "René Descartes and the Birth of Neuroscience," in *Decisions, Uncertainty, and the Brain: The Science of Neuroeconomics* (Cambridge: MIT Press, 2004), 17.

41. Walter Pagel and Pyarali Rattansi, "Vesalius and Paracelsus," *Medical History* 8, no. 4 (1964): 318, doi: 10.1017/S0025727300029781.

42. James O. Menzoian, "Ambroise Pare: Barber Vascular Surgeon," *Journal of Vascular Surgery* 68, no. 2 (2018): 647, doi: 10.1016/j.jvs/2018.04.053.

43. Menzoian, "Ambroise Pare: Barber Vascular Surgeon," 647.

44. Seymour J. Schwartz, *The Anatomist, the Barber-Surgeon, and the King: How the Accidental Death of Henry II of France Changed the World* (New York: Humanity Books, 2015), 94.

45. Schwartz, *Anatomist,* 136.

46. Michael J. North, "The Death of Andreas Vesalius," *Circulating Now* (2014), accessed October 2, 2018, https://circulatingnow.nlm.nih.gov/2014/10/15/the-death-of-andreas-vesalius.

47. North, "The Death of Andreas Vesalius."

48. Rowland Jackson, *A Physical Dissertation on Drowning: In Which Submersion, Commonly Call'd Drowning, Is Shewn to Be a Long Time Consistent with the Continuance of Life...* (London: Golden Lion, 1746), 6.

49. Jackson, *A Physical Dissertation on Drowning*, 6.

50. Erwin H. Ackerknect, *A Short History of Medicine* (Baltimore: Johns Hopkins University Press, 2016), 74.

Chapter 2

1. *News from Basing-Stoak, Of One Mrs. Blunden a Maltsters Wife, who was Buried Alive* (John Millet, 1680), 4.

2. *News from Basing-Stoak*, 6.

3. *News from Basing-Stoak*, 7.

4. *News from Basing-Stoak*, 8.

5. *News from Basing-Stoak*, 8.

6. Walter Scott, *The Works of Jonathan Swift: Miscellaneous Poems* (Edinburgh: Archibald Constable and Co., 1814), 96.

7. F.P. Wilson, *The Plague in Shakespeare's London* (Oxford: Oxford University Press, 1927), 24.

8. Richelle Munkhoff, "Searchers of the Dead: Authority, Marginality, and the Interpretation of Plague in England," *Gender & History* 11, no. 1 (1999): 25, doi: 10.1111/1468-0424.00127.

9. Her Majestie and Her Privie Counsell, *Orders Thought Meete* (London: Deputies of Christopher Barker, 1594).

10. Wilson, *Plague in Shakespeare's London*, 9.

11. Wilson, *Plague in Shakespeare's London*, 8.

12. Ben Jonson, *The Alchemist*, Act 5, Scene 5.1 (London, 1610; Project Gutenberg, 2013).

13. Her Majestie and Her Privie Counsell, *Orders Thought Meete*.

14. Her Majestie and Her Privie Counsell, *Orders Thought Meete*.

15. Wilson, *Plague in Shakespeare's London*, 114.

16. Worshipful Company of Parish Clerks, "A True Report of All of the Burials and Christenings… 1602-1603" (London: *Guildhall Library*, 1603). Eighteenth Century Collections Online.

17. Thomas Dekker, *The Wonderful Yeare. 1603. Where in shewed the picture of London, lying sicke of the Plague* (London: Thomas Creede, 1603), C4-5.

18. Thomas Dekker, *The Seven Deadly Sinnes of London: Drawn in Seven Several Coaches, Through the Seen Several Gates of the City; Bringing the Plague with Them [October] 1606* (London, 1879), 87.

19. Dekker, *Seven Deadly Sinnes*, 47.

20. Dekker, *Seven Deadly Sinnes*, 47.

21. Dekker, *Seven Deadly Sinnes*, 47.

22. John Donne, *XXVI. Sermons (Never Before Publish'd)* (London: Thomas Newcomb, 1661), 296.

23. Margaret DeLacy, "The Conceptualization of Influenza in Eighteenth-Century Britain: Specificity and Contagion," *Bulletin of the History of Medicine* 67, no. 1 (1993): 79.

24. United States Public Health Service, *Public Health Reports: Volume 38, Part 1, Numbers 1-26* (Washington, D.C.: Government Printing Office, 1923), 735.

25. Victor Robinson, *The Story of Medicine* (New York: The New Home Library, 1944), 310.

26. Nick Lane, "The Unseen World: Reflections on Leeuwenhoek (1677) 'Concerning Little Animales,'" *Philosophical Transactions of the Royal Society B* 370 (2015): 1. https://doi.org/10.1098/rstb.2014.0344.

27. Richard Mead, *A Short Discourse Concerning Pestilential Contagion: And the Methods to be used to Prevent it* (London: Sam. Buckley in Amen-Corner, 1720), 2.

28. Mead, *A Short Discourse Concerning Pestilential Contagion*, 3.

29. Howard Haggard, *Mystery, Magic, and Medicine* (New York: Doubleday, Doran, 1933), 68.

30. Haggard, *Mystery, Magic, and Medicine*, 69.

31. Robinson, *The Story of Medicine* (New York: The New Home Library, 1944), 291.

32. W. Bruce Fye, "Realdo Colombo," *Clinical Cardiology* 25 (2002): 136.

33. William Harvey, *On the Motion of the Heart and Blood in Animals* (London: George Bell and Sons, 1889), 50.

34. Harvey, *On the Motion of the Heart and Blood in Animals*, 72.

35. Stanley G. Schultz, "William Harvey and the Circulation of the Blood: The Birth of a Scientific Revolution and Modern Physiology," *News in Physiological Sciences* 17, no. 5 (2002): 177, https://doi.org/10.1152/nips.01391.2002.

36. Schultz, "William Harvey and the Circulation of the Blood…," 178.

37. Schultz, "William Harvey and the Circulation of the Blood…," 178.

38. Edited by Knut Boeser, *The Elixirs of Nostradamus: Nostradamus' Original recipes for Elixirs, Scented Water, Beauty Potions and Sweetmeats* (Wakefield: Moyer Bell, 1996), 5–6.

39. Benjamin Woolley, *Heal Thyself: Nicholas Culpeper and the Seventeenth-Century Struggle to Bring Medicine to the People* (New York: HarperCollins, 2004), 20.

40. P. Hunting, "The Worshipful Society of Apothecaries of London," *Postgrad Medical Journal* 80 (2004): 41.

41. Wayne Shumaker, *The Occult Sciences in the Renaissance* (Berkeley: University of California Press, 1973), 18.

42. Woolley, *Heal Thyself,* 123.

43. Bank of England, "Inflation Calculator," 2021, accessed June 9, 2021, https://www.bankofengland.co.uk/monetary-policy/inflation/inflation-calculator.

44. Woolley, *Heal Thyself,* 124.

45. Thomas Carlyle, *The Letters and Speeches of Oliver Cromwell* (London: Methuen & Co., 1904), 22.

46. Woolley, *Heal Thyself,* 125.

47. Woolley, *Heal Thyself,* 125.

48. Woolley, *Heal Thyself,* 125.

49. John A. Paris, *Medical Jurisprudence* (London: W. Phillips, 1823), 226.

50. Paris, *Medical Jurisprudence,* 227.

51. Woolley, *Heal Thyself,* 126.

52. Woolley, *Heal Thyself,* 130.

53. Woolley, *Heal Thyself,* 130.

54. Royal College of Physicians of London, *The Case of the College of Physicians London, Wherein They Are Defendants, in a Writ of Error Retornable in Parliament, Brought by One William Rose an Apothecary in London, on a Judgement obtained Against Him by the College in Her Majesty's Court of Queen's-Bench, for Practising Physick within Seven Miles of London Without Licence* (London, 1704), 2.

55. Harold J. Cook, *The Decline of the Old Medical Regime in Stuart London* (Ithaca: Cornell University Press, 1986), 96.

56. Woolley, *Heal Thyself,* 135.

57. Woolley, *Heal Thyself,* 162.

58. Woolley, *Heal Thyself,* 166.

59. Clare Gittings, *Death, Burial, and the Individual in Early Modern England* (London: Croom Helm, 2001), 7.

60. Woolley, *Heal Thyself,* 166.

61. Richard Mabey, *Weeds: How Vagabond Plants Gatecrashed Civilisation and Changed the Way We Think About Nature* (New York: HarperCollins, 2010), n.p.

62. Nicholas Culpeper, *Astrological Judgement of Diseases from the Decumbiture of the Sick...* (London: Golden Angel, 1665), title page. Reprinted 2003.

63. Harvey, "On the Motion of the Heart and Blood in Animals," 72.

64. *A Strange and Wonderfull Relation of the Burying Alive of Joan Bridges of Rochester in the County of Kent* (London, 1646), 4.

65. *Strange and Wonderfull Relation,* 4.

66. *Strange and Wonderfull Relation,* 4.

67. *The Most Lamentable and Deplorable Accident which on Friday last June 22. Befell Laurence Cawthorn a butcher in St. Nicholas Shambles in Newgate Market, who being suspected to be Dead, by the two hasty covetousness and cruelty of his Land-lady Mrs. Cook in Pincock-lane, was suddenly and inhumanely buryed* (London, 1661), 11.

68. *Most Lamentable and Deplorable Accident,* 12.

69. *Most Lamentable and Deplorable,* 13.

70. *Most Lamentable and Deplorable,* 16.

Chapter 3

1. "The Following Remarkable Circumstance Is Extracted from Dr. Cricton's Essay on Mental Derangement," *Chester Courant* (Chester, England), October 16, 1798. Accessed June 8, 2020. British Newspaper Archive.

2. "The Following Remarkable Circumstance Is Extracted from Dr. Cricton's Essay."

3. "The Following Remarkable Circumstance Is Extracted from Dr. Cricton's Essay."

4. Rosemary Horrox, "Purgatory, Prayer and the Plague: 1150–1380," in *Death in England: An Illustrated History,* ed. Peter Jupp and Clare Gittings (New Brunswick: Rutgers University Press, 2000), 93.

5. Horrox, "Purgatory, Prayer and the Plague: 1150–1380," 90.

6. John M. Theilmann, "The Miracles of King Henry VI of England," *Historian* 42, no. 3 (1980): 457.

7. Philip Morgan, "Of Worms and War: 1380–1558," in *Death in England: An Illustrated History,* ed. Peter Jupp and Clare Gittings (New Brunswick: Rutgers University Press, 2000), 131.

8. Ann Thomson, *Bodies of Thought: Science, Religion, and the Soul in the Early Enlightenment* (London: Oxford University Press), 167.

9. Thomson, *Bodies of Thought,* 42.

10. Thomson, *Bodies of Thought,* 42.

11. Thomson, *Bodies of Thought,* 42.

12. Gert-Jan Lokhorst, "Descartes and the Pineal Gland," *The Stanford Encyclopedia of Philosophy* (Winter 2018 edition), ed. Edward N. Zalta, accessed May 24, 2020. https://plato.stanford.edu/archives/win2018/entries/pineal-gland.

13. Lokhorst, "Descartes and the Pineal Gland."

14. Maria Pia Donato, "The Mechanical Medicine of a Pious Man of Science: G. M. Lancisi's *De subitaneis mortibus* (1707)," *Conflicting Duties: Science, Medicine and Religion in Rome 1550–1750,* eds. Jill Kraye and Maria Pia Donato (London: The Warburg Institute, 2009), 322.

15. Axel Karenberg, "Cerebral Localization in the Eighteenth Century—An Overview," *Journal of the History of the Neuroscience* 18 (2009): 249.

16. Donato, "The Mechanical Medicine of a Pious Man of Science," 346.

17. Donato, "The Mechanical Medicine of a Pious Man of Science," 347.

18. Rev. Donald J. Bretherton, "Lazarus of Bethany: Resurrection or Resuscitation?" *The Expository Times* 104, no. 6 (1993): 170.

19. Bretherton, "Lazarus of Bethany: Resurrection or Resuscitation?" 170.

20. Bretherton, "Lazarus of Bethany: Resurrection or Resuscitation?" 170.

21. Bretherton, "Lazarus of Bethany: Resurrection or Resuscitation?" 170.

22. Bretherton, "Lazarus of Bethany: Resurrection or Resuscitation?" 170.

23. John Marsh, *The Gospel of St. John* (Baltimore: Penguin Books, 1968), 438.

24. Bretherton, "Lazarus of Bethany: Resurrection or Resuscitation?" 171.

25. Bretherton, "Lazarus of Bethany: Resurrection or Resuscitation?" 171.

26. John Engelbrecht, *The German Lazarus; Being a Plain and Faithful Account of the Extraordinary Events That Happened to John Engelbrecht of Brunswick Relating to His Apparent Death, and Return to Life: With the Commission Give to Him During That Interval* (London: Ben Bragg, 1707), 2.

27. Engelbrecht, *German Lazarus,* 25.

28. Engelbrecht, *German Lazarus,* 26.

29. Engelbrecht, *German Lazarus,* 32.

30. Phillipe Ariès, *The Hour of Our Death* (Oxford: Oxford University Press, 1981), 356.

31. "London, March 28," *Stamford Mercury* (Lincolnshire, England), April 2, 1741. British Newspaper Archive.

32. A Society of Gentlemen in Scotland, *Encyclopaedia Britannica; or, a Dictionary of Arts and Sciences, Complied upon a New Plan* (Edinburgh: A. Bell and C. Macfarquhar, 1771), 309.

33. William Rider, *A New Universal English Dictionary or, A Compleat Treasure of the English Language* (Oxford: W. Griffin, 1759), np.

34. G.S. Plaut, "Dr. John Fothergill and Eighteenth-Century Medicine," *Journal of Medical Biography* 7 (1999): 192.

35. Robert Kilpatrick, "'Living in the Light' Dispensaries, Philanthropy and Medical Reform in Late-Eighteenth-Century London," in *The Medical Enlightenment of the Eighteenth Century,* ed. Andrew Cunningham and Roger French (Cambridge: Cambridge University Press, 2006), 260.

36. Kilpatrick, "'Living in the Light' Dispensaries, Philanthropy and Medical Reform in Late-Eighteenth-Century London," 260.

37. William Tossach, "A Man Dead in Appearance, Recovered by Distending the Lungs with Air," in *Medical Essays and Observations,* 4th ed. A Society in Edinburgh (Edinburgh: Hamilton, Balfour, and Neill, 1752), 109.

38. Tossach, "A Man Dead in Appearance," 111.

39. John Fothergill, *Observations on the Recovery of a Man Dead in Appearance* (London, 1745), 4–5.

40. Fothergill, *Observations on the Recovery of a Man Dead in Appearance,* 7.

41. Alexander Johnson, *Dr. Johnson's Abridged Instructions of Recovering Persons Apparently Dead* (London, 1785), 1.

42. Johnson, *Dr. Johnson's Abridged Instructions,* 1.

43. Johnson, *Dr. Johnson's Abridged Instructions*, 2.
44. Charles Kite, *An Essay on the Recovery of the Apparently Dead* (London: C. Dilly in the Poultry, 1788), 107–108.
45. Kite, *Essay on the Recovery*, 108.
46. Kite, *Essay on the Recovery*, 108.
47. Ana Graciela Alzaga, et al., "Charles Kite: The Clinical Epidemiology of Sudden Cardiac Death and the Origin of the Early Defibrillator," *Resuscitation* 62 (2005): 7.
48. James Curry, *Popular Observations on Apparent Death from Drowning, Suffocation, &c. with an Account of the Means to be Employed for Recovery* (London: Law and Son, 1792), B2.
49. Curry, *Popular Observations*, B2.
50. Curry, *Popular Observations*, 5.
51. Robert M. Sade, "Brain Death, Cardiac Death, and the Dead Donor Rule," *Journal of the South Carolina Medical Association* 107, no. 4 (2011): 146–149, https://www.ncbi.nlm.nih.gov/pmc/articles/PMC3372912.
52. Curry, *Popular Observations*, 2.
53. Curry, *Popular Observations*, 2.
54. A. Fothergill, *Preservation Plan, or Hints for the Preservation of Persons Exposed to Those Accidents Which Suddenly Suspend or Extinguish Vital Action, and by Which Many Valuable Lives Are Prematurely Lost to the Community* (London: H. L. Galabin, 1798), 21.
55. A. Fothergill, *Preservation Plan*, 40.
56. A. Fothergill, *Preservation Plan*, 22.
57. A. Fothergill, *Preservation Plan*, 41.
58. A. Fothergill, *Preservation Plan*, 42.
59. Walter Whiter, *A Dissertation on the Disorder of Death; Or That State of the Frame Under the Signs of Death Called Suspended Animation; to Which Remedies Have Been Sometimes Successfully Applied, as in other Disorders, in Which It Is Recommended, That the Same Remedies of Resuscitative Process Should be Applied to cases of NATURAL DEATH, As They Are to Cases of Violent Death, Drowning, &c. Under the Same Hope of Sometimes Succeeding in the Attempt* (Norwich, 1819), vi.
60. Whiter, *A Dissertation on the Disorder of Death*, 378.
61. Whiter, *A Dissertation on the Disorder of Death*, 17.
62. Whiter, *A Dissertation on the Disorder of Death*, 16.

63. Whiter, *A Dissertation on the Disorder of Death*, 443.
64. Whiter, *A Dissertation on the Disorder of Death*, 444.
65. Whiter, *A Dissertation on the Disorder of Death*, 444.
66. Elizabeth Stevens, "'Dead Eyes Open': The Role of Experiments in Galvanic Reanimation in Nineteenth-Century Popular Culture," *Leonardo* 48, no. 3 (2015), 276.
67. W. Hawes, *Royal Humane Society: Annual Report* (London: J. Nichols, 1798), 62.
68. Hawes, *Royal Humane Society: Annual Report*, 1798, 63.
69. "Galvanism," *Northampton Mercury* (Northampton, England), January 29, 1803. Held by the British Newspaper Archive.
70. Whiter, *A Dissertation on the Disorder of Death*, 41.
71. Whiter, *A Dissertation on the Disorder of Death*, 401.
72. James Cowles Prichard, *A Review of the Doctrine of a Vital Principle: As Maintained by Some Writers* (London: John and Arthur Arch, 1829), 17.
73. Prichard, *A Review of the Doctrine of a Vital Principle: As Maintained by Some Writers*, 18.
74. William Buchan, *Domestic Medicine; or the Family Physician: Being an Attempt to Render the Medical Art More Generally Useful, by Shewing People What Is in Their Own Power Both with Respect to the Prevention and Cure of Diseases* (Philadelphia: Joseph Crukshank, 1774), 443.
75. "A Definition of Irreversible Coma: Report of the Ad Hoc Committee of the Harvard Medical School to Examine the Definition of Brain Death," *JAMA* 22, no. 5 (1984): 678.
76. Anne L. Dalle Ave and James L. Bernat, "Inconsistencies Between the Criterion and Tests for Brain Death," *Journal of Intensive Care Medicine* 25, no. 8 (2020): 772.
77. Dalle Ave and Bernat, "Inconsistencies Between the Criterion," 773.
78. Dalle Ave and Bernat, "Inconsistencies Between the Criterion," 772.

Chapter 4

1. "Monday's Post: From the St. James's Evening-Post, March 12. Ireland. Dublin,

March 5," *Derby Mercury*, 1736. British Newspaper Archive, accessed October 18, 2018.

2. Seema K Shah, et al., "Death and Legal Fictions," *Journal of Medical Ethics* 37, no. 12 (2011): 720.

3. "For the Kentish Gazette," *Kentish Gazette*, 1789. British Newspaper Archive.

4. *Kentish Gazette*, 1789.

5. Jean-Benigne Winslow, *The Uncertainty of the Signs of Death and the Danger of Precipitate Interments and Dissections* (London: The Globe, 1746), 14.

6. Winslow, *Uncertainty of the Signs of Death*, 14.

7. Winslow, *Uncertainty of the Signs of Death*, 305. This edition published in Dublin, 1746, by George Faulkner.

8. William Tebb, *Premature Burial and How it may be Prevented* (London: Swan Sonnanschein & Co., 1905), 73–74.

9. Winslow, *The Uncertainty of the Signs of Death* (Dublin), 19.

10. Georges Leonetti, et al., "Evidence of Pin Implementation as a Means of Verifying Death During the Great Plague of Marseilles (1722)," *Journal of Forensic Science* 42, no. 4 (1997): 745.

11. John Bowden, *A Sermon on Job xxx.—23. Preach'd at the Funeral of Mr. James Blunt, of Frome on Thursday the 19th of August, 1749* (Bristol: Thomas Cadell, 1749), 8.

12. Bowden, *Sermon on Job xxx.—23*, 2–3.

13. Bowden, *Sermon on Job xxx.—23*, 4.

14. Bowden, *Sermon on Job xxx.—23*, 7.

15. Bowden, *Sermon on Job xxx.—23*, 6.

16. Alexander Johnson, *A Collection of Authentic Cases Proving the Practicability of Recovering Persons Visibly Dead by Drowning, Suffocation, Stifling, Swooning, Convulsions, and Other Accidents* (London: John Nourse, 1775), 126.

17. Erin O'Shea, "Horse, Warrior: Famous Residents of RAF Lakenheath," Royal Air Force Lakenheath, Royal Airforce Lakenheath, January 26, 2015, accessed April 12, 2021, https://www.lakenheath.af.mil/News/Article-Display/Article/727822/horse-warrior-famous-residents-of-raf-lakenheath.

18. O'Shea, "Horse, Warrior: Famous Residents of RAF Lakenheath."

19. Rosemary Horrox, "Purgatory, Prayer and the Plague: 1150–1380," in *Death*

in England: An Illustrated History, ed. Peter Jupp and Clare Gittings, 93.

20. Horrox, "Purgatory, Prayer and the Plague: 1150–1380," 93.

21. Vanessa Harding, "Burial of the Plague Dead in Early Modern London," *Epidemic Disease in London*, ed. J.A.I Champion (Center for Metropolitan History Working Papers Series) no. 1 (1993): 62.

22. Harding, "Burial of the Plague Dead in Early Modern London," 53.

23. Clare Gittings, *Death, Burial, and the Individual in Early Modern England* (London: Croom Helm, 2001), 47–48.

24. *A Directory for the Publique Worship of God Throughout the Three Kingdomes of England, Scotland, and Ireland* (London: T.R. & E.M, 1651), 49.

25. Clare Gittings, "Sacred and Secular: 1558–1660," in *Death in England: An Illustrated History*, ed. Peter Jupp and Clare Gittings (New Brunswick: Rutgers University Press, 2000), 150.

26. Gittings, "Sacred and Secular: 1558–1660," 150.

27. Ruth Richardson, *Death, Dissection, and the Destitute* (Chicago: University of Chicago Press, 2000), 19.

28. Richardson, *Death, Dissection, and the Destitute*, 20.

29. Clare Gittings, "Eccentric or Enlightened? Unusual Burial and Commemoration in England, 1689–1823," *Mortality* 12, no. 4 (2007): 326.

30. Richardson, *Death, Dissection, and the Destitute*, 23.

31. Ralph Houlbrooke, "The Age of Decency: 1660–1760," in *Death in England: An Illustrated History*, ed. Peter Jupp and Clare Gittings (New Brunswick: Rutgers University Press, 2000), 192.

32. Richardson, *Death, Dissection, and the Destitute*, 18.

33. Richardson, *Death, Dissection, and the Destitute*, 12.

34. Jens Amendt, et al., "Forensic Entomology in Germany," *Forensic Science International* 11 (2000): 310.

35. B.B. Dent, et al., "Review of Human Decomposition Processes in Soil," *Environmental Geology* 42, no. 4 (2004): 577.

36. "Case from Granger's History of England," *Ipswich Journal* (Suffolk, England), March 12, 1791. British Newspaper Archive.

37. "Thursday 04 October 1787," *Hereford Journal* (Herefordshire, England), 1787. British Newspaper Archive.

38. "Thursday 04 October 1787," *Hereford Journal*, 1787.

39. Winslow, *The Uncertainty of the Signs of Death* (London), 28.

40. Liza Picard, *Dr. Johnson's London: Coffee-Houses and Climbing Boys, Medicine, Toothpaste and Gin, Poverty and Press-Gangs, Freakshows and Female Education* (New York: St. Martin's Press, 2000), 75.

41. Houlbrooke, "The age of decency: 1660–1760," 193.

42. Richardson, *Death, Dissection, and the Destitute*, 57.

43. Bank of England, "Inflation Calculator," 2020, accessed June 1, 2021, https://www.bankofengland.co.uk/monetary-policy/inflation/inflation-calculator.

44. James Blake Bailey, *Diary of a Resurrectionist, 1811–1812* (London: Swan Sonnanschein & Co., 1896), 64.

45. Bank of England, "Inflation Calculator," 2020, accessed June 1, 2021, https://www.bankofengland.co.uk/monetary-policy/inflation/inflation-calculator.

46. Bailey, *Diary of a Resurrectionist, 1811–1812*, 16–17.

47. John Craig, *A New Universal Etymological and Pronouncing Dictionary of the English Language, Embracing all the Terms Used in Art, Science, and Literature* (London: Henry George Collins, 1848), np.

48. "London, Jan 23," *Sussex Advertiser* (Sussex, England), January 29, 1749. British Newspaper Archive.

49. "ADVERTISEMENT EXTRAORDINARY," *Morning Post* (London, England), October 29, 1811. British Library Newspapers, accessed April 30, 2020. Gale Document Number: GALE|R3209497897.

50. "Union Hall," *Hull Packet* (East Yorkshire, England), December 9, 1817. British Newspaper Archive.

51. "Night-Robbers, and Body-Snatchers," *Morning Advertiser* (London, England), October 27, 1818. British Newspaper Archive.

52. "Union-Hall," *Bristol Mirror* (Bristol, England), November 16, 1816. British Newspaper Archive.

53. "Union-Hall," *Bristol Mirror* (Bristol, England), November 16, 1816. British Newspaper Archive.

54. Bransby Blake Coope, *The Life of Sir Astley Cooper* (London: John W. Parker, 1868), 339.

Chapter 5

1. Joseph Taylor, *The Danger of Premature Interment, Proved from Many Remarkable Instances of People Who Have Recovered After Being Laid Out for Dead, and of Others Entombed Alive, for Want of Being Properly Examined Prior to Interment* (London: W. Simpkin and R. Marshall, 1816), 24.

2. Harold Ellis, "The Company of Barbers and Surgeons," *Journal of the Royal Society of Medicine* 94, no. 10 (2001), 549.

3. Helen McDonald, *Human Remains: Dissection and Its Histories* (New Haven: Yale University Press, 2005), 11.

4. McDonald, *Human Remains*, 12.

5. Anita Guerrini, "The Value of a Dead Body," in *Vital Matters: Eighteenth-Century Views of Conception, Life, and Death*, ed. Helen Deutsch and Mary Terrall (Toronto: University of Toronto Press, 2012), 247.

6. William Hunter, *Two Introductory Lectures, Delivered by Dr. William Hunter, to His Last Course of Anatomical Lectures, at his Theatre in Windmill-Street: As They Were Left Corrected for the Press by Himself* (London, 1784), 88.

7. Hunter, *Two Introductory Lectures, Delivered by Dr. William Hunter*, 88.

8. Hunter, *Two Introductory Lectures, Delivered by Dr. William Hunter*, 87.

9. Guerrini, "The Value of a Dead Body," 250.

10. Lord Hansard, "Schools of Anatomy," *Parliament* 9 (1831): 302, accessed November 27, 2018, https://api.parliament.uk/historic-hansard/commons/1831/dec/15/schools-of-anatomy#column_302.

11. Howard Haggard, *Mystery, Magic, and Medicine* (New York: Doubleday, Doran, 1933), 82.

12. Wendy Moore, *The Knife Man: Blood, Body Snatching, and the Birth of Modern Surgery* (New York: Broadway Books, 2005), 5.

13. Betsy C. Corner and Christopher C. Booth, *Chain of Friendship: Selected*

Letters of Dr. John Fothergill of London, 1735–1780 (Cambridge: Belknap Press of Harvard University Press, 1971), 13.

14. The House of Commons, *Report from the Select Committee on Anatomy* (London, 1828), 4.

15. The House of Commons, *Report from the Select Committee*, 4.

16. James Blake Bailey, *Diary of a Resurrectionist, 1811–1812* (London: Swan Sonnanschein & Co., 1896), 68.

17. William Tebb, *Premature Burial and How It May Be Prevented* (London: Swan Sonnanschein & Co., 1905), 379.

18. Copy of a Warrant of the President, Dr. Charles Goodall, to the Sheriffs of the City of London and Sheriff of the County of Middlesex, 1709, RCP-LEGAC/ENV 27, Royal College of Physicians of London.

19. Thomas W. Laqueur, *The Work of the Dead: A Cultural History of Mortal Remains* (Princeton: Princeton University Press, 2015), 149–150.

20. Laqueur, *The Work of the Dead*, 148.

21. Piers D. Mitchell, Ceridwen Boston, Andrew T. Chamberlain, et al., "The Study of Anatomy in England from 1700 to the Early 20th Century," *Journal of Anatomy* 219, no. 2 (2011): 94.

22. Mitchell et al., "The Study of Anatomy in England from 1700 to the Early 20th Century," 94.

23. Mitchell et al., "The Study of Anatomy in England from 1700 to the Early 20th Century," 94.

24. Anno 25, George II, c. 67. Parliamentary Archives.

25. Laqueur, *The Work of the Dead*, 337.

26. Elizabeth T. Hurren, "'Other Spaces' for the *Dangerous Dead* of Provincial England, c. 1752–1832," *Journal of the Historical Association* 103, no. 354 (2018): 29.

27. H.T. Dickinson, "Democracy," in *An Oxford Companion to the Romantic Age British Culture 1776–1832*, ed. Iain McCalman (Oxford: Oxford University Press, 1999), 35.

28. Ralph Houlbrooke, "The Age of Decency: 1660–1760," in *Death in England: An Illustrated History*, ed. Peter C. Jupp and Clare Gittings, 193.

29. Sarah Wise, *The Italian Boy: Murder and Grave-Robbery in 1830s London* (London, Jonathan Cape, 2004), 31; Richard Burn, *The Justice of the Peace, and Parish Officer* (London: A. Strahan, 1830), 353. Statute: *Rex v. Lynn, M. 1788, 2 T. R. 733.*

30. "Tuesday's Post," *Ipswich Journal* (Suffolk, England), July 1, 1786. British Newspaper Archive.

31. His Majesty's Justices Assigned to Keep the Peace within the County of Huntingdon, "Body Stealing: William Patrick and William Whayley, labourers of Farcet were Charged with Stealing from Yaxley Churchyard the Recently Interred Body of Jane Mason…," 1830, The Court in Session: Bundles, HCP, 1, 14, 3, p. 1, Huntingdonshire Archives.

32. Huntingdon Quarter Sessions Court, "The Court in Session: Bundles," 1830, HCP, 1, 1, 4. Huntingdonshire Archives.

33. Mitchell, et al., "The Study of Anatomy in England," 94.

34. Cooper, *The Life of Sir Astley Cooper*, 352.

35. "Resurrection Men," *Staffordshire Advertiser* (Stafford, England), December 31, 1796. British Newspaper Archive.

36. "Resurrection Men," *Staffordshire Advertiser*, December 31, 1796.

37. "Resurrection Men," *Staffordshire Advertiser*, December 31, 1796.

38. Cooper, *The Life of Sir Astley Cooper*, 350–351.

39. Cooper, *The Life of Sir Astley Cooper*, 351.

40. "Union Hall," *Hull Packet* (East Yorkshire, England), December 9, 1817. British Newspaper Archive.

41. "Inquests," *Public Ledger and Daily Advertiser* (London, England), October 15, 181, 4. British Newspaper Archive.

42. Cooper, *The Life of Sir Astley Cooper*, 340.

43. Thomas Hood, *The Complete Poetical Words of Thomas Hood* (London: Henry Frowde, 1906), 77.

44. Hood, *The Complete Poetical Words of Thomas Hood*, 77.

45. Robert Southey, *The Poetical Works of Robert Southey: Collected by Himself, Volume 6* (London: Longman, Orme, Brown, Green, & Longmans, 1838), 185.

46. Southey, *The Poetical Works of Robert Southey*, 186.

47. Southey, *The Poetical Works of Robert Southey*, 186.

48. Southey, *The Poetical Works of Robert Southey*, 186.

49. Southey, *The Poetical Works of Robert Southey*, 187.

50. John Knott, "Popular Attitudes to Death and Dissection in Early Nineteenth Century Britain: The Anatomy Act and the Poor," *Labour History* 49 (1985): 3.

51. Knott, "Popular Attitudes to Death and Dissection in Early Nineteenth Century Britain," 5.

52. The House of Commons, *Report from the Select Committee*, 9.

53. Knott, "Popular Attitudes to Death and Dissection in Early Nineteenth Century Britain," 6.

54. Rachel R. Hammer, Trahern W. Jones, Fareeda Taher Nazer Hussain, et al., "Students as Resurrectionists—A Multimodal Humanities Project in Anatomy Putting Ethics and Professionalism I Historical Context," *Anat Sci Educ* 3 (2010): 245. doi:10.1002/ase.174.

55. "Trial of the Burkers: Old Bailey.—(This Day.)," *London Courier and Evening Gazette* (London, England), December 2, 1831. British Newspaper Archive.

56. "Trial of the Burkers: Old Bailey.—(This Day.)," *London Courier and Evening Gazette*, December 2, 1831.

57. Wise, *The Italian Boy: Murder and Grave-Robbery in 1830s London*, 78.

58. Wise, *The Italian Boy: Murder and Grave-Robbery in 1830s London*, 196.

59. "Trial of the Burkers: Old Bailey.—(This Day.)," *London Courier and Evening Gazette*, December 2, 1831.

60. "Trial of the Burkers: Old Bailey.—(This Day.)," *London Courier and Evening Gazette*, December 2, 1831.

61. "Trial of the Burkers: Old Bailey.—(This Day.)," *London Courier and Evening Gazette*, December 2, 1831.

62. Wise, *The Italian Boy: Murder and Grave-Robbery in 1830s London*, 205.

63. Wise, *The Italian Boy: Murder and Grave-Robbery in 1830s London*, 205.

64. Bailey, *Diary of a Resurrectionist, 1811–1812*, 105.

65. "An Act for Regulating Schools of Anatomy," *The Lancet* 18, no. 471 (1832): 712.

66. "An Act for Regulating Schools of Anatomy," 713.

67. "An Act for Regulating Schools of Anatomy," 713.

68. "An Act for Regulating Schools of Anatomy," 713.

69. "An Act for Regulating Schools of Anatomy," 715.

70. Knott, "Popular Attitudes to Death and Dissection," 7.

71. Bailey, *The Diary of a Resurrectionist*, 55.

72. Knott, "Popular Attitudes to Death and Dissection," 8.

Chapter 6

1. "Intelligence Extraordinary," *Caledonian Mercury* (Edinburgh, Scotland), 1767. British Newspaper Archive.

2. Alexander Johnson, "A Short Account of a Society at Amsterdam," in *The Monthly Review, or Literary Journal From June 1773 to January 1774*, ed. Several Hands (London, 1774): 309.

3. "News," *Morning Chronicle* [1770] (London, England), December 3, 1773. *17th and 18th Century Burney Collection*. Gale Document Number: GALE|Z2000830261.

4. Johnson, "A Short Account of a Society at Amsterdam," 310.

5. Johnson, "A Short Account of a Society at Amsterdam," 311.

6. "Royal Humane Society: About Us," Royal Humane Society, accessed May 18, 2021, https://royalhumanesociety.org.uk/about-us/the-royal-humane-society.

7. Samuel Glasse, *Dr. Glasse's Sermon, in Favour of the Humane Society, March 17, 1793* (London: John Nichols, 1793), 20.

8. F. Bull, *Annual Proceedings of the Society for the Recovery of the Apparently Drowned* (London, 1774).

9. Raymond Crawfurd, "William Hawes and the Royal Humane Society," *The Lancet*, 183, no. 4731 (1914): 1286.

10. "News," *Times* (London, England), January 26, 1789. 17th and 18th Century Burney Collection. Gale Document Number: GALE|Z2001482062.

11. "News," *Morning Chronicle* [1770] (London, England), July 30, 1795. 17th and 18th Century Burney Collection. Gale Document Number: GALE|Z2000806604.

12. "News," *Morning Chronicle*, July 30, 1795.

13. William Hawes, *An Address to the King and Parliament of Great Britain on Preserving the Lives of the Inhabitants* (London: J. Dodsey, 1783), 6.

14. "News," *London Chronicle* (London, England), January 11, 1791–January 13, 1791. 17th and 18th Century Burney Collection. Gale Document Number: GALE|Z20005 93266.

15. Alexander Johnson, *Relief from Accidental Death; or, Summary Directions, in Verse, Extracted from the Instructions at Large* (London: Logographic Press, 1789), 10.

16. Johnson, *Relief From Accidental Death*, 6.

17. Johnson, *Relief From Accidental Death*, 7.

18. "Leeds," *Leeds Intelligencer* (Yorkshire, England), December 29, 1789. British Newspaper Archive.

19. Rev. W. Agutter, "Reflections on the Preservation of Life," *Northampton Mercury* (Northampton, England), May 18, 1793. British Newspaper Archive.

20. Agutter, "Reflections on the Preservation of Life," *Northampton Mercury* (Northampton, England).

21. Medline Plus, "CPR—Adult and Child After Onset of Puberty," U.S. National Library of Medicine, 2021, accessed June 11, 2021. https://medlineplus.gov/ency/article/000013.htm.

22. Alexis A. Topjian, et al., "Brain Resuscitation in the Drowning Victim," *Neurocrit Care* 17 (2012): 442, doi: 10.1007/s12028-012-9747-4.

23. Anthony J. Handley, "Drowning," *British Medical Journal* 348 (2014), https://doi.org/10.1136/bmj.g1734.

24. Ian Maconochie, et al., "Resuscitating Drowned Children," *British Medical Journal* 350, no. 104 (2015), 1. doi: 10.1136/bmj.h535.

25. Maconochie, et al., "Resuscitating Drowned Children," 1.

26. Maconochie, et al., "Resuscitating Drowned Children," 1.

27. Glasse, *Dr. Glasse's Sermon*, 24.

28. Glasse, *Dr. Glasse's Sermon*, 24.

29. John Snart, *Thesaurus of Horror; Or, the Charnel House Explored* (London: Sherwood, Neely, and Jones, 1817), 175.

30. Jan Bondeson, *Buried Alive: The Terrifying History of Our Most Primal Fear* (London: W.W. Norton, 2001), 240.

31. Bondeson, *Buried Alive*, 240.

32. B.B. Dent, et al., "Review of Human Decomposition Processes in Soil," *Environmental Geology* 45 (2004): 577.

Chapter 7

1. "Extract of a Letter from Paris, May 24," *Chelmsford Chronicle* (Essex, England), June 3, 1785. British Newspaper Archive.

2. "I. Italy," *Ipswich Journal* (Suffolk, England), April 15, 1749. British Newspaper Archive.

3. "London, July 23," *Newcastle Chronicle* (Northumberland, England), July 30, 1768. British Newspaper Archive.

4. "London, July 23," July 30, 1768.

5. "To the Printer," *Derby Mercury* (Derbyshire, England), June 16, 1791. Held by the British Newspaper Archive.

6. Amicus, "To the Printer," *Northampton Mercury* (Northampton, England), September 19, 1789. British Newspaper Archive.

7. "Singular Case," *Hampshire Chronicle* (Winchester, England), June 23, 1798. British Newspaper Archive.

8. "London," *Derby Mercury* (Derbyshire, England), May 3, 1733. British Newspaper Archive.

9. "London," *Derby Mercury* (Derbyshire, England), May 3, 1733. British Newspaper Archive.

10. Jan Bondeson, *Buried Alive: The Terrifying History of Our Most Primal Fear* (London: W.W. Norton, 2001), 119.

11. James Cocks, *Memorials of Hatherlow and of the old Chadkirk Chapel* (Stockport: Claye and Sons, 1895), 187.

12. Cocks, *Memorials of Hatherlow and of the old Chadkirk Chapel*, 187.

13. Christian H. Eisenbrandt, "Coffin to be used in cases of doubtful death," U.S. Patent 3335A, November 15, 1843. https://patents.google.com/patent/US3335A/en.

14. Serba Smith, "The Life Preserving Coffin," *The Columbian Magazine*, January 1844, 36.

15. Walter Whiter, *A Dissertation on the Disorder of Death; Or That State of the Frame Under the Signs of Death Called Suspended Animation; to Which Remedies Have Been Sometimes Successfully Applied, as in other Disorders, In Which It Is Recommended, That the Same Remedies of Resuscitative Process Should Be Applied to Cases of NATURAL DEATH, As They Are to Cases of Violent Death, Drowning, &c. Under the Same Hope of Sometimes Succeeding in the Attempt* (Norwich, 1819), 57.

16. Whiter, *A Dissertation on the Disorder of Death*, 65.

17. "Death Certificates Recommendations of the Committee," *Manchester Evening News* (Manchester, England), September 2, 1893. British Newspaper Archive.

18. "Death Certificates Recommendations of the Committee," *Manchester Evening News* (Manchester, England), September 2, 1893.

19. George K. Behlmer, "Grave Doubts: Victorian Medicine, Moral Panic, and the Signs of Death," *Journal of British Studies* 42, no. 2 (2003): 228.

20. William Tebb, *Premature Burial and How it may be Prevented* (London: Swan Sonnanschein & Co., 1905), 277–278.

21. Tebb, *Premature Burial*, 18.

22. David Walsh, *Premature Burial: Fact or Fiction* (London: Bailliere, Tindall and Cox, 1897), 5.

23. Walsh, *Premature Burial: Fact or Fiction*, 6.

24. Walsh, *Premature Burial: Fact or Fiction*, 7.

25. Walsh, *Premature Burial: Fact or Fiction*, 12.

26. Behlmer, "Grave Doubts," 225.

27. Tebb, *Premature Burial*, 8.

28. Walsh, *Premature Burial: Fact or Fiction*, 10–11.

29. Greg Kelly, "A Review of the History of Body Temperature and Its Variability Due to Site Selection, Biological Rhythms, Fitness, and Aging," *Alternative Medicine Review* 11, no. 4 (2006): 279.

30. Jas. R. Williamson, "Premature Burial," in *The Metaphysical Magazine: Volume IX* (New York: The Metaphysical Publishing Company, 1899), 319.

31. William Tebb and Col. Edward Perry Vollum, *Premature Burial and How It May Be Prevented* (London: Swan Sonnenschien & Co., 1896), 188.

32. Tebb, *Premature Burial and How it may be Prevented*, 194.

33. Charles Becker and Ken Darby, "Little Billy" Rhodes, et al, *The Wizard of Oz* (Hollywood: Metro Goldwyn Mayer, 1939), motion picture.

34. Meinhardt Raabe and Rad Robinson, *The Wizard of Oz* (Hollywood: Metro Goldwyn Mayer, 1939), motion picture.

Chapter 8

1. "Deaths," *Scots Magazine* (Midlothian, Scotland), February 1, 1785, 103. British Newspaper Archive.

2. Victor Turner, "Liminality and Communitas," in *The Ritual Process: Structure and Anti-Structure* (Chicago: Aldine Publishing, 1969), 359.

3. Turner, "Liminality and Communitas," 359.

4. Dariusz Błaszczyk, "Vampires from Drawsko," Foundation for Polish History and Culture, 2014, http://www.slavia.org/fieldschool.php?go=drawsko_vampires.

5. David Barrowclough, "Time to Slay Vampire Burials? The Archaeological and Historical Evidence for Vampires in Europe," *Red Dagger Press* (2014): 2.

6. Barrowclough, "Time to Slay Vampire Burials?" 1.

7. Christopher Daniell and Victoria Thompson, "Pagans and Christians: 400–1150," in *Death in England: An Illustrated History*, ed. Peter Jupp and Clare Gittings (New Brunswick: Rutgers University Press, 2000), 192.

8. Theresa Bane, *Encyclopedia of Vampire Mythology* (Jefferson: McFarland & Company, 2017), 13.

9. Bob Curran, "Was Dracula an Irishman?" *History Ireland* 8, no. 2 (2000): 12.

10. Bane, *Encyclopedia of Vampire Mythology*, 13.

11. Rachel Nuwer, ""Vampire Grave" in Bulgaria Holds a Skeleton with a Stake Through its Heart," *Smithsonian Magazine*, 2014, https://www.smithsonianmag.com/smart-news/vampire-grave-bulgaria-holds-skeleton-stake-through-its-heart-180953004.

12. Barrowclough, "Time to Slay Vampire Burials?" 3.

13. Barrowclough, "Time to Slay Vampire Burials?" 3.

14. Christine Dell'Amore, "'Vampire of Venice' Unmasked: Plague Victim & Witch?" *National Geographic*, 2010, https://www.nationalgeographic.com/news/2010/2/100226-vampires-venice-plague-skull-witches.

15. Stephen Gordon, "Social Monsters and the Walking Dead in William of Newburg's Historia Rerum Anglicarum," *Journal of Medieval History* 41, no. 4 (2015): 449.

16. David Keyworth, "Was the Vampire of the Eighteenth Century a Unique Type of Undead-Corpse?" *Folklore* 117, no. 3 (2006): 243.

17. Jacqueline Simpson, "Repentant Soul of Walking Corpse? Debatable Apparitions in Medieval England," *Folklore* 114 no. 3 (2003): 393.

18. Keyworth, "Was the Vampire of the Eighteenth Century a Unique Type of Undead-Corpse?" 243.

19. Keyworth, "Was the Vampire of the Eighteenth Century a Unique Type of Undead-Corpse?" 243.

20. Keyworth, "Was the Vampire of the Eighteenth Century a Unique Type of Undead-Corpse?" 244.

21. Samuel Taylor Coleridge, *Christabel, by Samuel Taylor Coleridge; Illustrated by a Facsimile of the Manuscript and by Textual and Other Notes, by Ernest Hartley Coleridge* (London: H. Frowde, 1907), 20.

22. Coleridge, *Christabel*, 29.

23. *The Lost Boys*, directed by Joel Schumacher (1987; Burbank: Warner Home Video, 1998), DVD.

24. Coleridge, *Christabel*, 69–70.

25. Coleridge, *Christabel*, 70.

26. James B. Twitchell, *The Living Dead: A Study of the Vampire in Romantic Literature* (Durham: Duke University Press, 1981), 40.

27. Rosemary Horrox, "Purgatory, Prayer and the Plague: 1150–1380," in *Death in England: An Illustrated History*, ed. Peter Jupp and Clare Gittings, 95.

28. Augustin Calmet, *The Phantom World: The History and Philosophy of Spirits, Apparitions, etc., etc. From the French of August Calmet*, translated by the Rev. Henry Christmas (Philadelphia: A. Hart, Late Carey & Hart, 1850), 2.

29. Stephen Gordon, "Emotional Practice and Bodily Performance in Early Modern Vampire Literature," *Preternature: Critical and Historical Studies on the Preternatural* 6, no. 1 (2017): 107.

30. Keyworth, "Was the Vampire of the Eighteenth Century a Unique Type of Undead-Corpse?" 248.

31. Keyworth, "Was the Vampire," 248.

32. Thomas Walsingham, *The Chronica Maiora of Thomas Walsingham, 1376–1422*, translated by David Preest (Suffolk: The Boydell Press, 2005), 301.

33. Calmet, *The Phantom World*, 52.

34. Calmet, *The Phantom World*, 52.

35. Calmet, *The Phantom World*, 52.

36. "One Evening Last Week I Call'd to See a Friend and…," *Country Journal, or the Craftsman* (London, England), May 20, 1732. 17th and 18th Century Nicholas Newspapers Collection. Gale Document Number: GALE|PGNHLS694164329.

37. "One Evening Last Week."

38. "One Evening Last Week."

39. Gordon, "Emotional Practice," 100.

40. Gordon, "Emotional Practice," 100.

41. "One Evening Last Week I Call'd to See a Friend and…," *Country Journal, or the Craftsman*, May 20, 1732.

42. "One Evening Last Week I Call'd to See a Friend and…," *Country Journal, or the Craftsman* May 20, 1732.

43. "Gentlemen and Ladies, I Think this Dispute May be Easily…," *Country Journal, or the Craftsman* (London, England), May 20, 1732. 17th and 18th Century Nicholas Newspapers Collection. Gale Document Number: GALE|DOSLAA 099763338.

44. "Gentlemen and Ladies, I Think This Dispute May Be Easily…," *Country Journal, or the Craftsman*, May 20, 1732.

45. "Gentlemen and Ladies."

46. "Gentlemen and Ladies."

47. Carol Bolton, "*Thalaba the Destroyer*: Southey's Nationalist 'Romance,'" *Romanticism on the Net* no. 32–33 (2003), https://doi.org/10.7202/009260ar.

48. Bolton, "*Thalaba the Destroyer*: Southey's Nationalist 'Romance.'"

49. Robert Southey, *Thalaba the Destroyer* (United Kingdom: John Duncombe and Company, 1838), 280.

50. Southey, *Thalaba the Destroyer*, 280–281.

51. Southey, *Thalaba the Destroyer*, 297.

52. Southey, *Thalaba the Destroyer*, 297.

53. Southey, *Thalaba the Destroyer*, 297.

54. Southey, *Thalaba the Destroyer*, 298.

55. Poetry Foundation, "Lord Byron (George Gordon): 1788–1824," *Poetry Foundation*, 2020, accessed August 1, 2020, www.poetryfoundation.org/poets/lord-byron.

56. Poetry Foundation, "Lord Byron."

57. Poetry Foundation, "Lord Byron."

58. Lord Byron, *The Giaour: A Fragment of a Turkish Tale* (London: Thomas Davison, Whitefriars, 1813), 37.

59. Byron, *The Giaour: A Fragment of a Turkish Tale*, 38.

60. Marc Collins Jenkins, *Vampire Forensics* (Washington, D.C.: National Geographic, 2010), 116.

61. Gordon, "Emotional Practice and Bodily Performance in Early Modern Vampire Literature," 105.

62. Augustin Calmet, *The Phantom World: The History and Philosophy of Spirits, Apparitions, etc., etc.* (Philadelphia: A. Hart, 1850), 249. Translated 1850. Originally published 1751.

63. David Keyworth, "The Aetiology of Vampires and Revenants: Theological Debate and Popular Belief," *Journal of Religious History* 34, no. 2. (2010): 167.

64. Calmet, *The Phantom World*, 262.

65. Calmet, *The Phantom World*, 263.

66. Calmet, *The Phantom World*, 263.

67. Błaszczyk, "Vampires from Drawsko," Foundation for Polish History and Culture, 2014. http://www.slavia.org/field school.php?go=drawsko_vampires.

68. Keyworth, "The Aetiology of Vampires and Revenants," 161.

69. Keyworth, "The Aetiology of Vampires and Revenants," 161.

70. "*From the* GENERAL EVENING POST, June 29," *Newcastle Courant* (Northumberland, England), July 8, 1738, British Newspaper Archive.

71. "*From the* GENERAL EVENING POST, June 29," *Newcastle Courant*, July 8, 1738.

72. "Bristol, April 1," *Reading Mercury and Oxford Gazette* (Oxfordshire, England), April 10, 1786, British Newspaper Archive.

73. Mary W. Shelley, *Frankenstein; or, The Modern Prometheus* (Boston and Cambridge: Sever, Francis, & Co., 1869), 60.

74. John Polidori, *The Vampyre: A Tale* (London: Sherwood, Neely, and Jones, 1819), xxii.

75. Polidori, *Vampyre*, 41–42.

76. Polidori, *Vampyre*, 48.

77. Polidori, *Vampyre*, 72.

78. Carol A. Senf, *The Vampire in Nineteenth Century Literature* (Madison: University of Wisconsin Press, 1988), 60.

79. Bram Stoker, *Dracula* (New York: Random House, 1897), 334.

80. Stoker, *Dracula*, 52.

81. Stoker, *Dracula*, 53.

82. Stoker, *Dracula*, 56.

83. Stoker, *Dracula*, 219.

84. Stoker, *Dracula*, 234.

85. Stoker, *Dracula*, 235–236.

Conclusion

1. Samuel Glasse, *Dr. Glasse's Sermon, in Favour of the Humane Society, March 17, 1793* (London: John Nichols, 1793), 22.

2. Edgar Allan Poe, *Works of Edgar Allan Poe* (Auckland: The Floating Press, 2014), 489.

Bibliography

Artwork

Illustrated Plate—The Signs of Death. 1746. Wellcome Collection, London, England. https://wellcomecollection.org/works/ag9g92sf.

A man supposed to be dead arising from his coffin and surprising his wife (?). Coloured aquatint, 1805, after a drawing by Henry Wigstead, 1784. Wellcome Collection, London, England. Attribution 4.0 International (CC BY 4.0). https://wellcomecollection.org/works/xxkcdgbr.

Morton, Erika. "MoD map—Salomone." 2020.

Salomone, Nicole. *Bunhill Fields Burial Grounds (London, England).* Photograph, 2019.

Salomone, Nicole. *Picture of Safety Coffin Alarm at Central Cemetery Museum (Vienna, Austria).* Photograph, 2018.

Smirke, Robert. *A man recuperating in bed at a receiving-house of the Royal Humane Society, after resuscitation by W. Hawes and J.C. Lettsom from near drowning.* Watercolour. Wellcome Collection, London, England. https://wellcomecollection.org/works/t6dcgvzq.

Vesalius, Andreas. *Fourth Muscle Man.* 1543.Wellcome Collection, London England. Attribution 4.0 International (CC BY 4.0).

Wigstead, Henry. *The dead alive!* 1784. Wellcome Collection, London, England. https://wellcomecollection.org/works/xxkcdgbr.

Primary Sources, Books

Buchan, William. *Domestic Medicine; or the Family Physician: Being an Attempt to Render the Medical Art More Generally Useful, by Shewing People What Is in Their Own Power Both with Respect to the Prevention and Cure of Diseases.* Philadelphia: Joseph Crukshank, 1774.

Bull, F. *Annual Proceedings of the Society for the Recovery of the Apparently Drowned.* London, 1774.

Burn, Richard. *The Justice of the Peace, and Parish Officer.* London: A. Strahan, 1830.

Curry, James. *Popular Observations on Apparent Death from Drowning, Suffocation, &c. with An Account of the Means to be Employed for Recovery.* London: Law and Son, 1792.

Dekker, Thomas. *The Seven Deadly Sinnes of London: Drawn in Seven Several Coaches, Through the Seen Several Gates of the City; Bringing the Plague with Them [October] 1606.* London, 1879.

Dekker, Thomas. *The Wonderful Yeare. 1603. Where in shewed the picture of London, lying sicke of the Plague.* London: Thomas Creede, 1603.

A Directory for the Publique Worship of God Throughout the Three Kingdomes of England, Scotland, and Ireland. London: T.R. & E.M, 1651.

Finch, Robert Pool. *A Sermon, Preached at Christ Church Middlesex, for the Benefit of the Humane Society.* London: John Nichols, 1788.

Fothergill, John. *Observations on the Recovery of a Man Dead in Appearance by Distending the Lungs with Air.* London, 1745.

Fothergill, A. *Preservation Plan, or Hints for the Preservation of Persons Exposed to Those Accidents Which Suddenly Suspend or Extinguish Vital Action, and by Which Many Valuable Lives are*

Prematurely Lost to the Community. London: H.L. Galabin, 1798.

Glasse, Samuel. *Dr. Glasse's Sermon, in Favour of the Humane Society, March 17, 1793.* London: John Nichols, 1793.

Graunt, John. *A Collection of the Yearly Bills of Mortality, From 1657 to 1758 Inclusive. Together with Several Other Bills of an Earlier Date.* London, 1759.

Harvey, William. *On the Motion of the Heart and Blood in Animals.* London: George Bell and Sons, 1889.

Hawes, W. *Royal Humane Society: Annual Report.* London: J. Nichols, 1798.

Hawes, William. *An Address to the King and Parliament of Great Britain on Preserving the Lives of the Inhabitants.* London: J. Dodsey, 1783.

Hawes, William. *Royal Humane Society Annual Report.* London: J. Nicholas, 1799.

Her Majestie and Her Privie Counsell. Orders Thought Meete. London: Deputies of Christopher Barker, 1594.

Hunter, William. *Two Introductory Lectures, Delivered by Dr. William Hunter, to his Last Course of Anatomical Lectures, at His Theatre in Windmill-Street: As They Were Left Corrected for the Press by Himself.* London, 1784.

Jackson, Rowland. *A Physical Dissertation on Drowning: In Which Submersion, Commonly Call'd Drowning, Is Shewn to be a Long Time Consistent with the Continuance of Life...* London: Golden Lion, 1746.

Johnson, Alexander. *An Address for Extending the Benefits of a Practice for Recovery from Accidental Death.* London, 1775.

Johnson, Alexander. *A Collection of Authentic Cases Proving the Practicability of Recovering Persons Visibly Dead by Drowning, Suffocation, Stifling, Swooning, Convulsions, and Other Accidents.* London: John Nourse, 1775.

Johnson, Alexander. *Dr. Johnson's Abridged Instructions of Recovering Persons Apparently Dead.* London, 1785.

Johnson, Alexander. *Relief from Accidental Death; or, Summary Directions, in Verse, Extracted from the Instructions at Large.* London: Logographic Press, 1789.

Kite, Charles. *An Essay on the Recovery of the Apparently Dead.* London: C. Dilly in the Poultry, 1788.

Mead, Richard. *A Short Discourse Concerning Pestilential Contagion: And the Methods to Be Used to Prevent it.* London: Sam. Buckley in Amen-Corner, 1720.

Paris, John A. *Medical Jurisprudence.* London: W. Phillips, 1823.

Prichard, James Cowles. *A Review of the Doctrine of a Vital Principle: As Maintained by Some Writers.* London: John and Arthur Arch, 1829.

Royal College of Physicians of London, *The Case of the College of Physicians London, Wherein They Are Defendants, in a Writ of Error Retornable in Parliament, Brought by One William Rose an Apothecary in London, on a Judgement Obtained Against Him by the College in Her Majesty's Court of Queen's-Bench, for Practising Physick Within Seven Miles of London Without Licence.* London, 1704.

Snart, John. *Thesaurus of Horror; Or, the Charnel House Explored.* London: Sherwood, Neely, and Jones, 1817.

Taylor, Joseph. *Apparitions: or, the Mystery of Ghosts, Hobgoblins, and Haunted Houses, Developed."* London: Lackington, Allen, and Co., 1815.

Taylor, Joseph. *The Danger of Premature Interment, Proved from Many Remarkable Instances of People Who Have Recovered After Being Laid out for Dead, and Others Entombed Alive, for Want of Being Properly Examined Prior to Interment.* London: W. Simpkin and R. Marshall, 1816.

Tebb, William. *Premature Burial and How it may be Prevented.* London: Swan Sonnanschein & Co., 1905.

Tebb, William; Vollum, Col. Edward Perry. *Premature Burial and How It May Be Prevented.* London: Swan Sonnenschien & Co., 1896.

Walsh, David. *Premature Burial: Fact or Fiction.* London: Bailliere, Tindall and Cox, 1897.

Whiter, Walter. *A Dissertation on the Disorder of Death; Or that State of the Frame Under the Signs of Death Called Suspended Animation; to Which Remedies Have Been Sometimes Successfully Applied, as in Other Disorders, In Which It Is Recommended, That the Same Remedies of Resuscitative Process Should Be Applied to Cases of NATURAL DEATH,*

As They Are to Cases of Violent Death, Drowning, &c. Under the Same Hope of Sometimes Succeeding in the Attempt. Norwich, 1819.

Williamson, Jas. R. "Premature Burial." in *The Metaphysical Magazine: Volume IX.* New York: The Metaphysical Publishing Company, 1899.

Primary Sources, Newspapers, Journals, Pamphlets, Laws, Legal Papers, etc.

"An Act Concerning Barbers and Surgeons to Be of One Company." Anno 32, Henry VIII, c. 42, 43. Parliamentary Archives.

"An Act for Regulating Schools of Anatomy." *The Lancet* 18 no. 471 (1832): 712–716.

ADVERTISEMENT EXTRAORDINARY." *Morning Post* (London, England), October 29, 1811. British Library Newspapers. Gale Document Number: GALE|R320 9497897.

Agutter, the Rev. W. "Reflections on the Preservation of Life." *Chester Chronicle* (Chester, England), April 5, 1793. British Newspaper Archive.

Agutter, the Rev. W. "Reflections on the Preservation of Life." *Northampton Mercury* (Northampton, England), May 18, 1793. British Newspaper Archive.

Amicus. "To the Printer." *Northampton Mercury* (Northampton, England), September 19, 1789. British Newspaper Archive.

Anno 25, George II, c. 67. Parliamentary Archives.

Bowden, John. *A Sermon on Job xxx.—23. Preach'd at the Funeral of Mr. James Blunt, of Frome on Thursday the 19th of August, 1749.* Bristol: Thomas Cadell, 1749.

"Bristol, April 1." *Reading Mercury and Oxford Gazette* (Oxfordshire, England), April 10, 1786. British Newspaper Archive.

"Case from Granger's History of England." *Ipswich Journal* (Suffolk, England), March 12, 1791. British Newspaper Archive.

Copy of a Warrant of the President, Dr. Charles Goodall, to the Sheriffs of the City of London and Sheriff of the County

of Middlesex or either of them to deliver of Middlesex or either of them to deliver unto the College Porter one body of a man or woman condemned and put to death. 1709. Royal College of Physicians of London: RCP-LEGAC/ENV 27.

"Death." *The Scots Magazine* (Midlothian, Scotland), February 1, 1785. British Newspaper Archive.

"Death Certificates Recommendations of the Committee." *Manchester Evening News* (Manchester, England), September 2, 1893. British Newspaper Archive.

"Edinburgh." *The Scots Magazine* (Edinburgh, Scotland), March 5, 1742, 44–45. British Newspaper Archive.

Eisenbrandt, Christian H. "Coffin to be used in cases of doubtful death." US Patent 3335A, November 15, 1843. https://patents.google.com/patent/US3335A/en.

Eisenbrandt, Christian Henry. "Life-Preserving Coffin; In Doubtful Cases of Actual Death." A61G17/02 Coffin closures; Packings therefor. 1843. https://patents.google.com/patent/US3335A/en.

Engelbrecht, John. *The German Lazarus; Being a Plain and Faithful Account of the Extraordinary Events That Happened to John Engelbrecht of Brunswick Relating to His Apparent Death, and Return to Life: With the Commission Give to Him During That Interval.* London: Ben Bragg, 1707.

"Extract of a letter from Paris, May 24." *Chelmsford Chronicle* (Essex, England), June 3, 1785. British Newspaper Archive.

"The Following Remarkable Circumstance Is Extracted from Dr. Cricton's Essay on Mental Derangement." *Chester Courant* (Chester, England), October 16, 1798. British Newspaper Archive.

"For the Kentish Gazette." *Kentish Gazette* (Kent, England), September 8, 1789. British Newspaper Archive.

"From the GENERAL EVENING POST, June 29." *Newcastle Courant* (Northumberland, England), July 8, 1738. British Newspaper Archive.

"Galvanism." *Northampton Mercury* (Northampton, England), January 29, 1803. Held by the British Newspaper Archive.

"Gentlemen and Ladies, I Think This Dispute May Be Easily..." *Country Journal,* or the *Craftsman* (London, England), May 20, 1732. 17th and 18th Century Nicholas Newspapers Collection. Gale Document Number: GALE| DOSLAA099763338.

His Majesty's Justices Assigned to Keep the Peace within the County of Huntingdon. "Body Stealing: William Patrick and William Whayley, labourers of Farcet were Charged with Stealing from Yaxley Churchyard the Recently Interred Body of Jane Mason..." 1830. The Court in Session: Bundles, HCP, 1, 14, 3. Huntingdonshire Archives.

The House of Commons. *Report from the Select Committee on Anatomy.* London, 1828.

Huntingdon Quarter Sessions Court, "The Court in Session: Bundles." 1830, HCP, 1, 1, 4. Huntingdonshire Archives.

"I. Italy." *Ipswich Journal* (Suffolk, England), April 15, 1749. British Newspaper Archive.

"Inquests." *Public Ledger and Daily Advertiser* (London, England). British Newspaper Archive.

"Intelligence Extraordinary." *Caledonian Mercury* (Suffolk, England), 1767. British Newspaper Archive.

Johnson, Alexander. "A Short Account of a Society at Amsterdam." *The Monthly Review, or Literary Journal From June 1773 to January 1774,* ed. Several Hands, 309–312. London, 1774.

Lane, Nick. "The Unseen World: Reflections on Leeuwenhoek (1677) 'Concerning Little Animals.'" *Philosophical Transactions of the Royal Society B* 370 (2015): 1–10. https://doi.org/10.1098/rstb.2014.0344.

"Leeds." *Leeds Intelligencer* (Yorkshire, England), December 29, 1789. British Newspaper Archive.

"London." *Derby Mercury* (Derbyshire, England), May 3, 1733. British Newspaper Archive.

"London, Jan 23." *Sussex Advertiser* (Sussex, England), January 29, 1749. British Newspaper Archive.

"London, July 23." *Newcastle Chronicle* (Northumberland, England), July 30, 1768. British Newspaper Archive.

"London Magazine. Means to Recover Persons Thought to Be Drowned." *The Scots Magazine* (Midlothian, Scotland), September 1745.

"London, March 28." *Stamford Mercury* (Lincolnshire, England), April 2, 1741. British Newspaper Archive.

"London, Tuesday, April 4." *Reading Mercury* (Berkshire, England), April 10, 1786. British Newspaper Archive.

"Monday's Post: From the St. James's Evening—Post, March 12. Ireland. Dublin, March 5." *Derby Mercury* (Derbyshire, England), 1736. British Newspaper Archive.

Money Laid Out for the College 24 May 1694 by John Cole (Bedell's Expenses) in Fetching a Dead Body from Tyburn for a College Dissection. 1694. Royal College of Physicians of London: RCP-LEGAC/ENV 27.

Money Paid Out by the College for Obtaining Dead Body from Tyburn 27 Feb 1694. 1694. Royal College of Physicians of London: RCP-LEGAC/ENV 27.

The Most Lamentable and Deplorable Accident which on Friday last June 22. Befell Laurence Cawthron a bucher in St. Nicholas Shambles in Newgate Market, who being suspected to be Dead, by the two hasty covetousness and cruelty of his Land-lady Mrs. Cook in Pincock-lane, was suddenly and inhumanely buryed. London, 1661.

"The Murder of the Italian Boy." *Morning Advertiser* (London, England), November 26, 1831. British Newspaper Archive.

"The Murdered Italian Boy." *Sussex Advertiser* (Sussex, England), November 28, 1831. British Newspaper Archive.

"News." *London Chronicle* (London, England), January 11, 1791–January 13 1791. 17th and 18th Century Burney Collection. Gale Document Number: GALE|Z2000593266.

"News." *Morning Chronicle* [1770] (London, England), December 3, 1773. 17th and 18th Century Burney Collection. Gale Document Number: GALE|Z2000830261.

"News." *Morning Chronicle* [1770] (London, England), January 23, 1777. 17th and 18th Century Burney Collection. Gale Document Number: GALE|Z2000844138.

"News." *Morning Chronicle* [1770] (London, England), July 30, 1795. 17th and 18th Century Burney Collection. Gale Document Number: GALE|Z2000806604.

"News." *Times* (London, England), January 26, 1789. 17th and 18th Century

Burney Collection. Gale Document Number: GALE|Z2001482062.

News from Basing-Stoak, of One Mrs. Blunden a Maltsters Wife, Who Was Buried Alive. John Millet, 1680.

"Night-Robbers, and Body-Snatchers." *Morning Advertiser* (London, England), October 27, 1818. British Newspaper Archive.

"On Vampires and Vampirism." *The New Monthly Magazine and Universal Register* 14, no. 82 (1820): 548–552.

"One Evening Last Week I Call'd to See a Friend and..." *Country Journal, or the Craftsman* (London, England), May 20 1732. 17th and 18th Century Nicholas Newspapers Collection. Gale Document Number: GALE|PGNHLS694164329.

"Resurrection Men." *Staffordshire Advertiser* (Stafford, England), December 31, 1796. British Newspaper Archive.

Robinson, Victor. *The Story of Medicine*. New York: The New Home Library, 1944.

Royal College of Physicians. "Dead Bodies: Petition of R.C.P to the House of Commons for Bill to Make Prevision for Redress in Matter of College Obtaining Executed Bodies for Dissection." 18th c?. Envelope 55, p. 68. Cat of Legal Docs, 1, Royal College of Physicians, London.

"Saturday 15 April 1749." *Ipswich Journal*, 1749. British Newspaper Archive.

"Singular Case." *Hampshire Chronicle* (Winchester, England), June 23, 1798. British Newspaper Archive.

"Singular Case." *Staffordshire Advertiser* (Staffordshire, England), June 23, 1798. British Newspaper Archive.

Smith, Serba. "The Life Preserving Coffin." *The Columbian Magazine*, January 1844.

A Society of Gentlemen in Scotland. *Encyclopaedia Britannica; or, a Dictionary of Arts and Sciences, Complied upon a New Plan*. Edinburgh: A. Bell and C. Macfarquhar, 1771.

Spriggs, John. "Body-Stealing: John Spriggs, New Town, Peterborough, Victualler, Disposed to Going, on Information Received from Weston, to the Hovel, and to the Removal of the Corpse to his Brewhouse." Huntingdonshire Archives: Huntingdonshire Quarter Sessions Records. HCP/1/14/10.

A Strange and wonderfull RELATION of The burying alive of Joan Bridges of Rochester in the County of Kent. London, 1646.

"Thursday 04 October 1787." *Hereford Journal* (Herefordshire, England), 1787. British Newspaper Archive.

"To the Printer." *Derby Mercury* (Derbyshire, England), June 16, 1791. British Newspaper Archive.

Tossach, William. "A Man Dead in Appearance, Recovered by Distending the Lungs with Air." in *Medical Essays and Observations*, 4th ed. A Society in Edinburgh. Edinburgh: Hamilton, Balfour, and Neill, 1752.

"Trial of the Burkers: Old Bailey.—(This Day)." *London Courier and Evening Gazette* (London, England). British Newspaper Archive.

"Tuesday's Post." *Ipswich Journal* (Suffolk, England), July 1, 1786. British Newspaper Archive.

"Union-Hall." *Bristol Mirror* (Bristol, England), November 16, 1816. British Newspaper Archive.

"Union Hall." *Hull Packet* (East Yorkshire, England), December 9, 1817. British Newspaper Archive.

Whayley, William. "Body-Stealing: Whayley, in a Long Statement Deposed to Being Persuaded to Dig up the Corpse of Jane Mason...." Huntingdonshire Archives: Huntingdonshire Quarterly Session Records. HCP/1/14/4.

"Wonderful Escape of a Sailor from Being Buried Alive." *Times* (London, England), Oct.16, 1788. *The Times Digital Archive*. Gale Document Number: GALE|CS67372880.

Worshipful Company of Parish Clerks. "A True Report of All of the Burials and Christenings... 1602–1603." London: Guildhall Library, 1603. Eighteenth Century Collections Online.

Secondary Sources

"About the Wellcome Osteological Research Database." Museum of London. Last modified 2018. https://www.museumoflondon.org.uk/collections/other-collection-databases-and-libraries/centre-human-bioarchaeology.

Ackerknect, Erwin H. *A Short History of Medicine*. Baltimore: Johns Hopkins University Press, 2016.

Aggarwal, Ankur. "The Evolving Relationship Between Surgery and Medicine." *American Medical Association Journal of Ethics* 12, no. 2 (2010): 119–123. doi: 10.1001/virtualmentor.2010.12.2.mhst1-1002.

Alzaga, Ana Graciela, Joseph Varon, and Peter Baskett. "Charles Kite: The Clinical Epidemiology of Sudden Cardiac Death and the Origin of the Early Defibrillator." *Resuscitation* 62, no. 1 (2005): 7–12.

Amendt, Jens, Roman Krettek, Constanze Niess, Richard Zehner, and Hansjurgen Bratzke. "Forensic Entomology in Germany." *Forensic Science International* 11 (2000): 309–314.

Apuleius. *Apuleii Opera Omnia ex Editione Oudendorpiana cum Notis et Interpretatione in Usum Delphini Variis Lectionibus Notis Variorum Recensu Editionus et Codicumet Indicibus Locupletissimis Accurate Recensita.* London: A.J. Valpy, AM, 1825.

Apuleius, Lucius. *The Apologia and Florida of Apuleius of Madaura.* Translated by H.E. Butler. Oxford: Clarendon Press, 1909; Kindle: Good Press, 2019.

Ariès, Phillipe. *The Hour of Our Death.* Oxford: Oxford University Press, 1981.

Arikha, Noga. *Passions and Tempers: A History of the Humours.* New York: HarperCollins, 2007.

Bailey, James Blake. *Diary of a Resurrectionist (1811–1812).* London: Swan Sonnanschein, & Co., 1896.

Bane, Theresa. *Encyclopedia of Vampire Mythology.* Jefferson: McFarland, 2017.

Bank of England. "Inflation Calculator." 2021. https://www.bankofengland.co.uk/monetary-policy/inflation/inflation-calculator.

Barclay, Andrew. *Electing Cromwell: The Making of a Politician.* London: Pickering & Chatto Limited, 2011.

Barrowclough, David. "Time to Slay Vampire Burials? The Archaeological and Historical Evidence for Vampires in Europe." *Red Dagger Press* (2014): 1–10.

Becker, Charles, Ken Darby, "Little Billy" Rhodes, et al. *The Wizard of Oz.* Hollywood: Metro Goldwyn Mayer, 1939, motion picture.

Behlmer, George K. "Grave Doubts: Victorian Medicine, Moral Panic, and the Signs of Death." *Journal of British Studies* 42, no. 2 (2003): 206–235.

Beyer, Jürgen. *Lay Prophets in Lutheran Europe (c. 1550–1700).* Leiden-Boston: Brill, 2017.

Błaszczyk, Dariusz. "Vampires from Drawsko." Foundation for Polish History and Culture, 2014. http://www.slavia.org/fieldschool.php?go=drawsko_vampires.

Boeser, Knut, ed. *The Elixirs of Nostradamus: Nostradamus' Original recipes for Elixirs, Scented Water, Beauty Potions and Sweetmeats.* Wakefield: Moyer Bell, 1996.

Bolton, Carol. "*Thalaba the Destroyer*: Southey's Nationalist "Romance." *Romanticism on the Net* no. 32–33 (2003). https://doi.org/10.7202/009260ar.

Bondeson, Jan. *Buried Alive: The Terrifying History of Our Most Primal Fear.* London: W.W. Norton, 2001.

Borzelleca, Joseph F. "Paracelsus: Herald of Modern Toxicology." *Toxicological Sciences* 53, no. 1 (2000): 2–4.

Boyacioglu Elif. "The Revenant on the Threshold." *Estonian Literary Museum Scholarly Press* 62 (2015): 7–36.

Boynton, Holmes, ed. *The Beginnings of Modern Science: Scientific Writings of the 16th, 17th, and 18th Centuries.* Roslyn: Walter J. Black, 1948.

Bretherton, Rev. Donald J. "Lazarus of Bethany: Resurrection or Resuscitation?" *The Expository Times* 104, no. 6 (1993): 169–173.

Buzwell, Greg. "Mary Shelley, *Frankenstein* and the Villa Diodati." British Library. Last modified May 15, 2014. https://www.bl.uk/romantics-and-victorians/articles/mary-shelley-frankenstein-and-the-villa-diodati.

Caciola, Nancy. "Wraiths, Revenants and Ritual in Medieval Culture." *Past & Present* no.152 (1996): 3–45.

Calmet, August. *The Phantom World: The History and Philosophy of Spirits, Apparitions, etc., etc. From the French of August Calmet.* Translated by the Rev. Henry Christmas. Philadelphia: A. Hart, Late Carey & Hart, 1850.

Calmet, Augustin. *The Phantom World: The History and Philosophy of Spirits, Apparitions, etc., etc.* Philadelphia: A. Hart, 1850. Translated 1850. Originally published 1751.

Carlyle, Thomas. *The Letters and Speeches*

of Oliver Cromwell. London: Methuen & Co., 1904.

Celsus, Aulus Cornelius. *A Literal Interlineal Translation of the First Four Books of Celsus De Medicina: With "Ordo" And Text: Tr. from the Text Selected for the Examination of Candidates At Apothecaries' Hall, And Other Public Boards; In Which the Elliptical Constructions Are Completed by Supplying the Suppressed Words, Shewing the Relations And Concords of the Different Words With Each Other*, 2d ed. Translated by Robert Venables. London: Sherwood, Gilbert, and Piper, 1837.

Clarke, Bob. *From Grub Street to Fleet Street: An Illustrated History of English Newspapers to 1899*. Brighton: Revel Barker Publishing, 2010.

Cocks, James. *Memorials of Hatherlow and of the old Chadkirk Chapel*. Stockport: Claye and Sons, 1895.

Coleridge, Samuel Taylor. *Christabel, by Samuel Taylor Coleridge; Illustrated by a Facsimile of the Manuscript and by Textual and Other Notes, by Ernest Hartley Coleridge*. London: H. Frowde, 1907.

Cook, Harold J. *The Decline of the Old Medical Regime in Stuart London*. Ithaca: Cornell University Press, 1986.

Cook, Harold J. "Good Advice and Little Medicine: The Professional Authority of Early Modern English Physicians." *Journal of British Studies* 33, no. 1 (1994): 1–31.

Cooper, Bransby Blake. *The Life of Sir Astley Cooper*. London: John W. Parker, 1868.

Copeman, W.S.C. "The Evolution of Anatomy and Surgery Under the Tudors." *Thomas Vicary Lecture Delivered at the Royal College of Surgeons of England* (1962): 1–21.

Corner, Betsy C., and Christopher C. Booth. *Chain of Friendship: Selected Letters of Dr. John Fothergill of London, 1735–1780*. Cambridge: Belknap Press of Harvard University Press, 1971.

Craig, John. *A New Universal Etymological and Pronouncing Dictionary of the English Language, Embracing All the Terms Used in Art, Science, and Literature*. London: Henry George Collins, 1848.

Crawfurd, Raymond. "William Hawes and

the Royal Humane Society." *The Lancet* 183, no. 4731 (1914): 1233–1298.

Culpeper, Nicholas. *Astrological Judgement of Diseases from the Decumbiture of the Sick...* London: Golden Angel, 1665. Reprinted 2003.

Cummins, Neil, Morgan Kelly, Cormac Ó Gráda. "Living Standards and Plague in London, 1560–1665." *Economic History Review* 69, no. 1 (2016): 3–34.

Curran, Bob. "Was Dracula an Irishman?" *History Ireland* 8, no. 2 (2000): 12–15.

"Currency converter: 1270–2017." The National Archives. Last modified 2018. https://www.nationalarchives.gov.uk/currency-converter.

Dalle Ave, Anne L., and James L. Bernat. "Inconsistencies Between the Criterion and Tests for Brain Death." *Journal of Intensive Care Medicine* 25, no. 8 (2020): 772–780.

Dalton, J.C. *Galen and Hippocrates*. New York: D. Appleton, 1873.

Daniell, Christopher, and Victoria Thompson. "Pagans and Christians: 400–1150." in *Death in England: An Illustrated History*, ed. Peter Jupp and Clare Gittings. New Brunswick: Rutgers University Press, 2000.

"A Definition of Irreversible Coma: Report of the Ad Hoc Committee of the Harvard Medical School to Examine the Definition of Brain Death." *JAMA* 22, no. 5 (1984).

DeLacy, Margaret. "The Conceptualization of Influenza in Eighteenth-Century Britain: Specificity and Contagion." *Bulletin of the History of Medicine* 67, no. 1 (1993): 74–118.

DeLacy, Margaret. *The Germ of an Idea*. New York: Palgrave Macmillian, 2016.

Dell'Amore, Christine. "'Vampire of Venice' Unmasked: Plague Victim & Witch?" National Geographic, 2010. https://www.nationalgeographic.com/news/2010/2/100226-vampires-venice-plague-skull-witches.

Dent, B.B., S.L. Forbes, and B.H. Stuart. "Review of Human Decomposition Processes in Soil." *Environmental Geology* 42, no. 4 (2004): 576–585.

Dickinson, H.T. "Democracy." in *An Oxford Companion to the Romantic Age British Culture 1776–1832*, ed. Iain McCalman. Oxford: Oxford University Press, 1999.

Dobson, MJ. "Malaria in England: A Geographical and Historical Perspective." *Parassitologia* 36 no. 1–2 (1994): 35–60. PMID: 7898959.

Donato, Maria Pia. "The Mechanical Medicine of a Pious Man of Science: G. M. Lancisi's *De subitaneis mortibus* (1707)." In *Conflicting Duties: Science, Medicine and Religion in Rome 1550–1750.* Jill Kraye and Maria Pia Donato, eds. London: The Warburg Institute, 2009.

Edward Worth Library. "Infectious Diseases: Theories of Contagion." *Edward Worth Library* (2020). http://infectiousdiseases.edwardworthlibrary.ie/Theory-of-Contagion.

Ellis, Harold. "The Company of Barbers and Surgeons." *Journal of the Royal Society of Medicine* 94, no. 10 (2001): 548–549. PMIC: PMC1282221.

Frank, Julia Bess. "Body Snatching: A Grave Medical Problem." *The Yale Journal of Biology and Medicine* 49 (1976): 399–410.

Fye, W.B. "Giovanna Maria Lancisi, 1654–1720." *Clinical Cardiology* 13 (1990): 670–671.

Fye, W. Bruce. "Realdo Colombo." *Clinical Cardiology* 24 (2002): 135–137.

Gardner-Nix, Jackie, Lucie Costin-Hall, and Jon Kabat-Zinn. *The Mindfulness Solution to Pain: Step-by-Step Techniques for Chronic Pain Management.* Oakland: Jackie Gardner-Nix, 2009.

Gibson, Susannah. *Animal, Vegetable, Mineral? How Eighteenth-Century Science Disrupted the Natural Order.* Oxford: Oxford University Press, 2015.

Gittings, Clare. *Death, Burial, and the Individual in Early Modern England.* London: Croom Helm, 2001.

Gittings, Clare. "Eccentric or enlightened? Unusual burial and commemoration in England, 1689–1823." *Mortality* 12, no. 4 (2007): 321–346.

Gittings, Clare. "Sacred and Secular: 1558–1660." In *Death in England: An Illustrated History,* Peter Jupp and Clare Gittings, eds. New Brunswick: Rutgers University Press, 2000.

Glimcher, Paul W. "René Descartes and the Birth of Neuroscience." In *Decisions, Uncertainty, and the Brain: The Science of Neuroeconomics.* Cambridge: MIT Press, 2004.

Goodwin, Gordon. "Kite, Charles (bap. 1760?, d. 1811), Surgeon." Oxford Dictionary of National Biography. Last Modified 2004. https://doi.org/10.1093/ref:odnb/15692.

Gordon, Stephen. "Emotional Practice and Bodily Performance in Early Modern Vampire Literature." *Preternature: Critical and Historical Studies on the Preternatural* 6, no. 1 (2017): 93–124.

Gordon, Stephen. "Social Monsters and the Walking Dead in William of Newburgh's *Historia Rerum Anglicarum.*" *Journal of Medieval History* 41, no. 4 (2015): 446–465.

Greenbaum, Dorian Giesler. "Astronomy, Astrology, and Medicine." *Handbook of Archaeoastronomy and Ethnoastronomy* (2014): 117–132. https://doi.org/10.1007/978-1-4614-6141-8_19.

Guerrini, Anita. "The Value of a Dead Body." In *Vital Matters: Eighteenth-Century Views of Conception, Life, and Death,* Helen Deutsch and Mary Terrall, eds., 246–264. Toronto: University of Toronto Press, 2012.

Haggard, Howard. *Mystery, Magic, and Medicine.* New York: Doubleday, Doran, 1933.

Hammer, Rachel R., Trahern W. Jones, Fareeda Taher Nazer Hussain, et al. "Students as Resurrectionists—A Multimodal Humanities Project in Anatomy Putting Ethics and Professionalism I Historical Context." *Anat Sci Educ* 3 (2010): 244–248. doi:10.1002/ase.174.

Handley, Anthony J. "Drowning." *British Medical Journal* 348 (2014). https://doi.org/10.1136/bmj.g1734.

Hannay, David. *A Short History of the Royal Navy 1217–1815, Volume II 1685–1815.* London: Methuen & Co., 2019.

Harding, Vanessa "Burial of the Plague Dead in Early Modern London." In *Epidemic Disease in London,* ed. J.A.I Champion (Center for Metropolitan History Working Papers Series) no. 1 (1993).

Hippocrates. "On Ancient Medicine." MIT: The Internet Classics Archive, Part 1. Translated by Francis Adams. Accessed December 11, 2017. http://classics.mit.edu/Hippocrates/ancimed.html.

Hippocrates. "On Ancient Medicine." MIT: The Internet Classics Archive, Part 5. Translated by Francis Adams. Accessed December 11, 2017. http://classics.mit.edu/Hippocrates/ancimed.html.

"The History of the Society." Royal Humane Society. Accessed June 22, 2018. https://www.royalhumanesociety.org.uk.

Hood, Thomas. *The Complete Poetical Words of Thomas Hood.* London: Henry Frowde, 1906.

Horrox, Rosemary. "Purgatory, Prayer and the Plague: 1150–1380." In *Death in England: An Illustrated History,* ed. Peter Jupp and Clare Gittings. New Brunswick: Rutgers University Press, 2000.

Houlbrooke, Ralph. "The Age of Decency: 1660–1760." In *Death in England: An Illustrated History,* ed. Peter Jupp and Clare Gittings, 174–201. New Brunswick: Rutgers University Press, 2000.

Huntin, P. "The Worshipful Society of Apothecaries of London." *Postgrad Medical Journal* 80 (2004): 41–44.

Hurren, Elizabeth T. *Dissecting the Criminal Corpse: Staging Post-Execution Punishment in Early Modern England.* London: Palgrave Macmillan, 2016.

Hurren, Elizabeth T. "'Other Spaces' for the *Dangerous Dead* of Provincial England, c. 1752–1832." *Journal of the Historical Association* 103, no. 354 (2018): 27–59.

Hutchison, Richard L., Rayan, Ghazi M. "Astley Cooper: His Life and Surgical Contributions." *History of Hand Surgery* 36, no. 2 (2011): 316–320. https://doi.org/10.1016/j.jhsa.2010.10.036.

Jenkins, Marc Collins. *Vampire Forensics.* Washington, D.C.: National Geographic, 2010.

Jonson, Ben. *The Alchemist.* Act 5, Scene 5.1. London, 1610; Project Gutenberg, 2013.

Karenberg, Axel. "Cerebral Localization in the Eighteenth Century—An Overview." *Journal of the History of the Neuroscience* 18 (2009): 248–253.

Katz, Arnold M., and Phillis B. Katz. "Diseases of the Heart in the Works of Hippocrates." *British Cardiovascular Society: Heart* 24 (1962): 257–264.

Kelly, Greg. "A Review of the History of Body Temperature and its Variability Due to Site Selection, Biological Rhythms, Fitness, and Aging." *Alternative Medicine Review* 11, no. 4 (2006): 278–293.

Keyworth, David. "The Aetiology of Vampires and Revenants: Theological Debate and Popular Belief." *Journal of Religious History* 34, no. 2 (2010): 158–173.

Keyworth, David. "Was the Vampire of the Eighteenth Century a Unique Type of Undead-Corpse?" *Folklore* 117, no. 3 (2006): 241–260.

Kilpatrick, Robert. "'Living in the Light' Dispensaries, Philanthropy and Medical Reform in Late-Eighteenth-Century London." In *The Medical Enlightenment of the Eighteenth Century,* ed. Andrew Cunningham and Roger French. Cambridge: Cambridge University Press, 2006.

Kirby, Peter. "A Short Statistical Sketch of the Child Labour Market I Mid-Nineteenth Century London." *French Journal of British Studies* XII, no. 3 (2003): 1–17.

Knott, John. "Popular Attitudes to Death and Dissection in Early Nineteenth Century Britain: The Anatomy Act and the Poor." *Labour History* 49 (1985): 1–18.

Koch, Philippa. "Experience and the Soul in Eighteenth-Century Medicine." *Church History* 83, no. 3 (2016): 552–586.

Kurath, Sherman M., ed. *Middle English Dictionary.* Ann Arbor: University of Michigan Press, 1998.

Laqueur, Thomas W. *The Work of the Dead: A Cultural History of Mortal Remains.* Princeton: Princeton University Press, 2015.

Laurenza, Domenico. "Art and Anatomy in Renaissance Italy: Images from a Scientific Revolution." *Metropolitan Museum of Art Bulletin* 69, no. 3 (2012): 5–48.

Leonetti, Georges, Michael Signoli, Anne Laure Pelissier, Pierre Champsaur, Israel Hershkovitz, Christian Brunet, and Olivier Dutour. "Evidence of Pin Implementation as a Means of Verifying Death During the Great Plague of Marseilles (1722)." *Journal of Forensic Science* 42, no. 4 (1997): 744–748.

Lokhorst, Gert-Jan. "Descartes and the Pineal Gland." *The Stanford Encyclopedia of Philosophy* (Winter 2018 edition), Edward N. Zalta, ed. Accessed May 24, 2020. https://plato.stanford.edu/archives/win2018/entries/pineal-gland.

Lord Byron. *The Giaour: A Fragment of A Turkish Tale.* London: Thomas Davison, Whitefriars, 1813.

Lord Hansard. "Schools of Anatomy." *Parliament* 9 (1831): 300–307. Accessed November 27, 2018. https://api.parliament. uk/historic-hansard/commons/1831/ dec/15/schools-of-anatomy#column_ 302.

Mabey, Richard. *Weeds: How Vagabond Plants Gatecrashed Civilisation and Changed the Way We Think About Nature.* New York: HarperCollins, 2010.

Mackowiak, Phillip A., Steven S. Wasserman, and Myron M. Levine. "A Critical Appraisal of 98.6oF, the Upper Limit of the Normal Body Temperature, and Other Legacies of Carl Reinhold August Wunderlich." *JAMA* 268, no. 12 (1992). PMID: 1302471.

Maconochie, Ian, and Charles D. Deakin. "Resuscitating Drowned Children." *British Medical Journal* 350, no. 104 (2015). doi: 10.1136/bmj.h535.

Malomo, A.O., O.E. Idowu, & F.C. Osuagwu. "Lessons from History: Human Anatomy, from the Origin to the Renaissance." *International Journal of Morphology* 24, no. 1 (2006): 99–104.

Mann, W.N. *Hippocratic Writings.* Translated by J. Chadwick. Harmondsworth: Penguin,1983.

Marsh, Jan. "Health & Medicine in the 19th Century." Victoria and Albert Museum. Last modified 2016. http://www.vam. ac.uk/content/articles/h/health-and-medicine-in-the-19th-century.

Marsh, John. *The Gospel of St. John.* Baltimore: Penguin, 1968.

Marshall, Peter. *Beliefs and the Dead in Reformation England.* Oxford: Oxford University Press, 2004.

McCraken-Flesher, Carol. *The Doctor Dissected: A Cultural Autopsy of the Bure & Hare Murders.* Oxford: Oxford University Press, 2012.

McDonald, Helen. *Human Remains: Dissection and Its Histories.* New Haven: Yale University Press, 2005.

McGavin, William. *The History of the Reformation of Religion in Scotland by John Knox; to Which Are Appended, Several Other Pieces of Hist Writing; Including the First Book of Discipline, Complete and His Dispute with the Abbot of Crossraguel, Not Given with Any Former Edition, with a Memoir, Historical Introduction, and Notes.* Glasgow: Blackie, Fullarton, & Co., 1831.

Medline Plus. "CPR—Adult and Child After Onst of Puberty." U.S. National Library of Medicine, 2021. https:// medlineplus.gov/ency/article/000013. htm.

Menzoian, James O. "Ambroise Pare: Barber Vascular Surgeon." *Journal of Vascular Surgery* 68, no. 2 (2018): 646–649. doi: 10.1016/j/jvs/2018.04.053.

Mitchell, Piers D., Ceridwen Boston, Andrew T. Chamberlain, Simon Chaplin, Vin Chauhan, Jonathan Evans, Louise Fowler, et al. "The Study of Anatomy in England from 1700 to the Early 20th Century." *Journal of Anatomy* 219, no. 2 (2011): 91–99.

Moore, Wendy. *The Knife Man: Blood, Body Snatching, and the Birth of Modern Surgery.* New York: Broadway Books, 2005.

Morgan, Philip. "Of Worms and War: 1380–1558." In *Death in England: An Illustrated History,* ed. Peter Jupp and Clare Gittings. New Brunswick: Rutgers University Press, 2000.

Morris, Leon. *The Gospel According to John.* Grand Rapids: Wm. B. Eerdmans, 1971.

Munkhoff, Richelle. "Searchers of the Dead: Authority, Marginality, and the Interpretation of Plague in England." *Gender & History* 11, no. 1 (1999), 1–29. doi: 10.1111/1468-0424.00127.

National Archives. "Currency Converter: 1270–2017." 2020. https://www.national archives.gov.uk/currency-converter.

National Library of Medicine. "Emotions and disease: The Balance of Passions." National Library of Medicine. Last modified May 2, 2012. https://www.nlm. nih.gov/exhibition/emotions/balance. html.

National Library of Medicine. "The World of Shakespeare's Humors." The National Library of Medicine. Last modified September 19, 2013. https://www.nlm. nih.gov/exhibition/shakespeare/four humors.html.

North, Michael J. "The Death of Andreas Vesalius." *Circulating Now,* 2014. https:// circulatingnow.nlm.nih.gov/2014/10/15/ the-death-of-andreas-vesalius.

Nutton, Vivian. "The Seeds of Disease: An Explanation of Contagion and Infection from the Greeks to the Renaissance." *Medical History* 27 (1983), 1–34.

Nuwer, Rachel. "'Vampire Grave' in Bulgaria Holds a Skeleton with a Stake Through Its Heart." *Smithsonian Magazine*, 2014. https://www.smithsonian mag.com/smart-news/vampire-grave-bulgaria-holds-skeleton-stake-through-its-heart-180953004.

Nye, Eric W. "Pounds Sterling to Dollars: Historical Conversion of Currency." Accessed August 28, 2018. http://www.uwyo.edu/numimage/currency.htm.

Ogilvie, Brian W. *The Science of Describing: Natural History in Renaissance Europe*. Chicago: University of Chicago Press, 2006.

O'Shea, Erin. "Horse, Warrior: Famous Residents of RAF Lakenheath." Royal Air Force Lakenheath, Royal Airforce Lakenheath, January 26, 2015. Accessed April 12, 2021. https://www.lakenheath. af.mil/News/Article-Display/Article/727822/horse-warrior-famous-residents-of-raf-lakenheath.

Pagel, Walter. *Paracelsus: An Introduction to Philosophical Medicine in the Era of the Renaissance*. New York: S. Karger, 1982.

Pagel, Walter, and Marianne Winder. "Harvey and the "Modern" Concept of Disease." *Bulletin of the History of Medicine* 42, no. 6 (1968): 496–509.

Pagel, Walter, and Pyarali Rattansi. "Vesalius and Paracelsus." *Medical History* 8, no. 4 (1964): 309–328. doi: 10.1017/S0025727300029781.

Park, Katharine. "The Criminal and the Saintly Body: Autopsy and Dissection in Renaissance Italy." *Renaissance Quarterly* 47, no. 1 (1994): 1–33.

Patel, Samir. "Plague Vampire Exorcism." Archeology Archive, 2009. https://archive.archaeology.org/online/features/halloween/plague.html.

Pearce, J.M.S. "John Fothergill: A Biographical Sketch and His Contributions to Neurology." *Journal of the History of Neurosciences* 22 (2013): 261–276.

Pernick, Martin. "Back from the Grave: Recurring Controversies Over Defining and Diagnosing Death in History." In *Death: Beyond Whole-Brain Criteria*, edited by Richard M. Zaner, 17–74. Dordrecht: Springer Netherlands, 1988.

Picard, Liza. *Dr. Johnson's London: Coffee-Houses and Climbing Boys, Medicine, Toothpaste and Gin, Poverty and Press-Gangs, Freakshows and Female Edu-cation*. New York: St. Martin's Press, 2000.

Plato. *Selected Dialogues of Plato: The Benjamin Jowett Translation, Revised and with an Introduction by Hayden Pelliccia*. New York: The Modern Library, 2001.

Plaut, G.S. "Dr. John Fothergill and Eighteenth-Century Medicine." *Journal of Medical Biography* 7 (1999): 192–196.

Poe, Edgar Allan. *Works of Edgar Allan Poe*. Auckland: The Floating Press, 2014.

Poetry Foundation. "Lord Byron (George Gordon): 1788–1824." *Poetry Foundation*, 2020. www.poetryfoundation.org/poets/lord-byron.

Poetry Foundation. "Robert Southey: 1774–1843." *Poetry Foundation*, 2020. www.poetryfoundation.org/poets/robert-southey.

Polidori, John. *The Vampyre: A Tale*. London: Sherwood, Neely, and Jones, 1819.

Raabe, Meinhardt; Robinson, Rad. *The Wizard of Oz*. Hollywood: Metro Goldwyn Mayer, 1939, motion picture.

Rees, Abraham. *The Cyclopaedia; Or, Universal Dictionary of Arts, Sciences and Literature*. United Kingdom: Longman, Hurst, 1819.

Richardson, Ruth. *Death, Dissection, and the Destitute*. Chicago: University of Chicago Press, 2000.

Rider, William. *A New Universal English Dictionary or, A Compleat Treasure of the English Language*. Oxford: W. Griffin, 1759.

Robinson, Victor. *Medicine in the 17th and 18th Century*. Whitefish: Kessinger, 2007.

Rosenberg, Charles E. "Medical Text and Social Context: Explaining William Buchan's 'Domestic Medicine.'" *Bulletin of the History of Medicine* 57, no 1 (1983): 22–42.

Ross, Ian, and Carol Urquhart Ross. "Body Snatching in Nineteenth Century Britain: From Exhumation to Murder." *British Society of Law and Society* 6, no. 1 (1979): 108–118.

Royal College of Physicians. "History of the Royal College of Physicians." Royal College of Physicians, 2020. https://www.rcplondon.ac.uk/about-us/who-we-are/history-royal-college-physicians.

Royal College of Physicians. "William Harvey." Royal College of Physicians,

2020. https://history.rcplondon.ac.uk/inspiring-physicians/william-harvey.

Royal Humane Society, and Robert M. Sad. "Brain Death, Cardiac Death, and the Dead Donor Rule." *Journal of the South Carolina Medical Association* 107, no. 4 (2011): 146–149. https://www.ncbi.nlm.nih.gov/pmc/articles/PMC3372912.

"Royal Humane Society: About Us." Royal Humane Society. Accessed August 31, 2018. https://www.royalhumanesociety.org.uk/about-us.

Schultz, Stanley G. "William Harvey and the Circulation of the Blood: The Birth of a Scientific Revolution and Modern Physiology." *News in Physiological Sciences* 17, no. 5 (2002): 175–180. https://doi.org/10.1152/nips.01391.2002.

Schumacher, Joel, dir. *The Lost Boys*. 1987. Burbank: Warner Home Video, 1998, DVD.

Schwartz, Seymour J. *The Anatomist, the Barber-Surgeon, and the King: How the Accidental Death of Henry II of France Changed the World*. New York: Humanity Books, 2015.

Scott, Walter. *The Works of Jonathan Swift: Miscellaneous Poems*. Edinburgh: Archibald Constable and Co., 1814.

Senf, Carol A. *The Vampire in Nineteenth Century Literature*. Madison: University of Wisconsin Press, 1988.

Shah, Seema K., Robert D. Truog, and Franklin G. Miller. "Death and Legal Fictions." *Journal of Medical Ethics* 37, no. 12 (2011): 719–722.

Shelley, Mary W. *Frankenstein; or, The Modern Prometheus*. Boston: Sever, Francis, & Co., 1869.

Shumaker, Wayne. *The Occult Sciences in the Renaissance*. Berkeley: University of California Press, 1973.

Simpson, Jacqueline. "Repentant Soul of Walking Corpse? Debatable Apparitions in Medieval England." *Folklore* 114, no. 3 (2003): 389–402.

Singal, R., R.P. Singal, A. Mittal, S. Sangwan, and N. Gupta. "Sir Astley Paston Cooper: History, English Surgeon and Anatomist." *Indian J Surg* 73, no 1 (2011): 82–84. doi:10.1007/s12262-010-0177-2.

Skal, David J. *Something in the Blood: The Untold Story of Bram Stoker, the Man Who Wrote Dracula*. New York: W.W. Norton, 2016.

Southey, Robert. *The Poetical Works of Robert Southey: Collected by Himself, Volume 6*. London: Longman, Orme, Brown, Green, & Longmans, 1838.

Southey, Robert. *Thalaba the Destroyer*. United Kingdom: John Duncombe and Company, 1838.

Stevens, Elizabeth. "'Dead Eyes Open': The Role of Experiments in Galvanic Reanimation in Nineteenth-Century Popular Culture." *Leonardo* 48, no. 3 (2015): 267–277.

Stoker, Bram. *Dracula*. New York: Random House, 1897.

Tersei, Dick. *The Undead: Organ Harvesting, the Ice-Water Test, Beating Heart Cadavers—How Medicine Is Blurring the Line Between Life and Death*. New York: Pantheon, 2012.

Theilmann, John M. "The Miracles of King Henry VI of England." *Historian* 42, no. 3 (1980): 456–471.

Thompson, C.J.S. "The Apothecary in England from the Thirteenth to the Close of the Sixteenth Century." *Proc R Soc Med* 8 (1915): 36–44.

Thomson, Ann. *Bodies of Thought: Science, Religion, and the Soul in the Early Enlightenment*. London: Oxford University Press, 2008.

Topjian, Alexis A., Robert A. Berg, Joost J.L.M. Bierens, Christine M. Branche, Robert S. Clark, Hans Friberg, Cornelia W.E. Hoedemaekers, et al. "Brain Resuscitation in the Drowning Victim." *Neurocrit Care* 17 (2012): 441–467. https://www.ncbi.nlm.nih.gov/pmc/articles/PMC3677166.

"Trial of John Bishop, Thomas Williams, and James May." Old Bailey Proceedings Online. December 1831. T18311201-17. www.oldbaileyonline.org.

Tristam, Kate. "Saint Cuthbert of Lindisfarne: The Body of Cuthbert: 635AD–687AD." The Holy Island of Lindisfarne. Accessed May 30, 2020. https://www.lindisfarne.org.uk/general/cuthbert2.htm.

Turner, Raphael. *Essentials of Microbiology*. EDTECH, 2018. E-book.

Turner, Victor. "Liminality and Communitas." In *The Ritual Process: Structure and Anti-Structure*. Chicago: Aldine, 1969, 94–113, 125–30. Abridged.

Twigg, Graham. "Plague in London: Spatial and Temporal Aspects of Mortality." *Epidemic Disease in London*, ed.

J.A.I. Champion (Centre for Metropolitan History Working Papers Series), no. 1 (1993): 1–17.

Twitchell, James B. *The Living Dead: A Study of the Vampire in Romantic Literature.* Durham: Duke University Press, 1981.

"Types of Brain Disorders: Anoxic & Hypoxic Brain Injury." Synapse, 2018. http://synapse.org.au/information-services/anoxic-hypoxic-brain-injury.aspx.

Underwood, Richard H. "Notes from the Underground (Sometimes Aboveground, Too)." *Savannah Law Review* 3, no. 1 (2016): 161–184.

United States Public Health Service. *Public Health Reports: Volume 38, Part 1, Numbers 1–26.* Washington, D.C.: Government Printing Office, 1923.

von Honenheim (Paracelsus), Theophrastus. *Volumen Medicinae Paramirum.* Baltimore: The Johns Hopkins Press, 1949. Translated from the original German by Kurt F. Leidecker, MA, PhD.

Walsingham, Thomas. *The Chronica Maiora of Thomas Walsingham, 1376–1422.* Translated by David Preest. Suffolk: The Boydell Press, 2005.

WebMD. "Anatomy and Circulation of the Heart." *WebMD,* 2020. https://www.webmd.com/heart-disease/high-cholesterol-healthy-heart#2.

Weir, Peter, dir. *Master and Commander.* 2003. Los Angeles: Twentieth Century Fox, DVD.

Wernerian Club, ed. *Pliny's Natural History* in *Thirty-Seven Books. A Translation on the Basis of That by Dr. Philemon Holland, Ed. 1601. With Critical and Explanatory Notes.* London: George Barclay, 1847–48, Book VII.

"William Hunter." University of Glasgow. Last modified 2018. https://www.universitystory.gla.ac.uk/biography/?id=WH0015&type=P.

Williams, Carolyn D. "Johnson, Alexander (bap. 1716, d. 1799), Physician and Advocate of Resuscitation." *Oxford Dictionary of National Biography.* Last modified 2004. https://doi.org/10.1093/ref:odnb/57457.

Wilson, FP. *The Plague in Shakespeare's London.* Oxford: Oxford University Press, 1927.

Winslow, Jaques-Benigne. *The Uncertainty of the Signs of Death.* Dublin: George Faulkner, 1746.

Winslow, Jean-Benigne. *The Uncertainty of the Signs of Death and the Danger of Precipitate Interments and Dissections.* London: The Globe, 1746.

Wise, Sarah. *The Italian Boy: Murder and Grave-Robbery in 1830s London.* London: Jonathan Cape, 2004.

Woolley, Benjamin. *Heal Thyself: Nicholas Culpeper and the Seventeenth-Century Struggle to Bring Medicine to the People.* New York: HarperCollins, 2004.

Zuckerman, Arnold. "Plague and Contagionism in Eighteenth-Century England: The Role of Richard Mead." *Bulletin of the History of Medicine* 78, no. 2 (2004): 273–308.

Index

Numbers in **bold italics** refer to pages with illustrations